WORLD PHILOSOPHY

THE SCEPTICAEMIC SURGEON

HOW NOT TO WIN FRIENDS AND INFLUENCE PEOPLE

WORLD PHILOSOPHY

Additional books in this series can be found on Nova's website under the Series tab.

Additional e-books in this series can be found on Nova's website under the e-book tab.

WORLD PHILOSOPHY

THE SCEPTICAEMIC SURGEON

HOW NOT TO WIN FRIENDS AND INFLUENCE PEOPLE

A COLLECTION OF ESSAYS
BY
MICHAEL BAUM

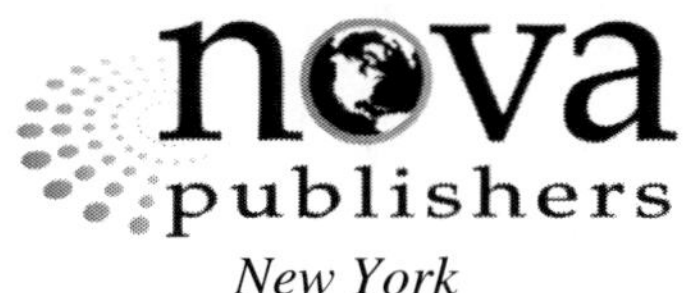

New York

Additional color graphics may be available in the e-book version of this book.

Library of Congress Cataloging-in-Publication Data

The scepticaemic surgeon : how not to win friends and influence people / editors, Michael Baum (Professor Emeritus of Surgery & Visiting Professor in Medical Humanities, University College London, UK).
pages cm. -- (World philosophy)
pages cm
ISBN 978-1-63463-050-4 (hardcover)
ISBN 978-1-63485-117-6 (softcover)
1. Medical ethics. I. Baum, Michael, 1937- editor.
R724.S3925 2014
174.2--dc23
2014036536

Published by Nova Science Publishers, Inc. † New York

Contents

Foreword

Clifford Hudis, MD
Chief, Breast Medicine Service and Attending Physician,
Memorial Sloan Kettering Cancer Center
Professor of Medicine, Weill Medical College of Cornell University
New York, NY, US
11 July 2014

When my old friend (and you can take that any way you please) Michael Baum emailed me with a request to pen – well, "keyboard" just doesn't have the same ring does it? – a brief forward to a collection of his writings, I was surprised. I am well aware of his creative skills, having had my dramatic debut on a big stage (and small audience) in Barcelona many years ago during the first production of his not-really-a-smash-hit show, "2084". Similarly, I knew well his propensity to speak his mind, firmly, precisely, and rationally, especially in the name of protecting the unknowing and vulnerable among us and without fear of power or authority. Turning to the 300 page pdf file he kindly provided – because I don't already have more than enough reading and writing to fill the day – I found that the chapter titles alone made for an amusing few minutes. Then I dug in. I spent the length of a flight to Asia reading these chapters and only then did I realize how prolific a writer he has been over the length of his career. He has written with zeal and with zingers. But always with humanity, humility and the best of intentions.

Friends and professional acquaintances will enjoy this book. They will flash back to lectures the attended and remember when Michael uttered the exact phrases now appearing in print. More importantly, they will feel the stir of emotion, passion, and maybe even anger, as the carefully constructed writing of a gifted communicator reminds them of the really big issues we have debated. That is not to say that others, including those of us not engaged in science and medicine, should stay away. For them, this book is a bit like one of those reality shows that try to show the general public what "really" goes on in the emergency room or hospital. Professor Baum shows the reader what is going on in his mind and that is the most informative and enlightening disclosure one could ever hope to experience.

From the first pages, one sees from his recollection of childhood exactly why he became what we learn about through his writings. The roots of his passion for justice, his thirst for knowledge, and his drive to simply set the world right were clearly present from his earliest days. Then, he turns to more granular expositions on society, science (focusing on breast cancer), and the influence of religion, leaders, and politicians. Throughout the book one is forced to stop and think carefully about widely held assumptions and dogma, not just in the traditional scientific realms but in the broader world as well. What emerged, for me, is an example of how to lead by example, respectfully question authority, be part of the solution rather than the problem, and to enjoy oneself along the way.

Professor Baum subtitled his book "how not to win friends and influence people". But that, too, is a tweak or a tease. He has in fact done exactly what he says these stories won't do. He has won friends and influenced a great many people. If any of us are lucky enough to be able to emulate his great example, we can only hope to accomplish half as much.

Preface

When you wish to grow bacteria in a Petrie dish it is important to select the right culture medium. Unfortunately for me I was implanted into a culture medium that favored the development of a progressive *"scepticaemia"* in later life. I grew up in an English orthodox Jewish household that has served to confuse my American colleagues because I speak "British" (with a posh plummy accent) but think "Yiddish". Us Yiddish thinkers are a contrary bunch. Almost from birth we are taught to see things from two perspectives at the same time: "on the one hand but on the other hand". In my family it was even more extreme. I was one of five siblings that belonged to two synagogues, one orthodox /orthodox and the other conservative/orthodox so at any one time one of us could argue that they wouldn't be seen dead in the other one's favored house of prayer. Friday night dinners always ended in a shouting match between four opinionated young men and one (the youngest) sister with our father the patriarch trying to keep order at the head of the table whilst our mother looked on indulgently from the kitchen as she ladled out the chicken soup. However whenever the conversation shifted to Israel and the Palestinians my father would join in with a vengeance. Like virtually all Jews of our acquaintance in those days we were all Zionists but in our family opinions raged between the secular right and left wings of the movement and the religious right and left wings of the movement. My position shifted because I was the contrarian and would side with whoever was losing the argument. Mind you my mother could also be a contrarian. There is the apocryphal story that she gave my oldest brother two ties for his 11th birthday. When he got dressed for synagogue the following Saturday he put on the red tie and when he proudly presented himself to our mother she responded by saying, "So what's wrong with the blue tie?"

Along with this behaviour trait we were all of a scientific frame of mind. My father, like many of his generation who fled the Russian pogroms, had no education but could play exhibition simultaneous chess taking on all comers, 12 boards at a time. He also played contract bridge for the City of Birmingham. My oldest brother, Geoffrey, was the first in the family to go to University and qualified as a doctor in 1951. My next brother, Harold, became professor of biochemistry and then Dean of life sciences at Kings College London and my youngest brother became professor of Paediatrics and Child Health at Bristol University and from there President of the Royal College of Paediatrics and Child Health in London. My young sister is still serving the National Health Service running a department of speech and language therapy. The next generation has already spawned three new professors in the life sciences. This toxic brew of religious orthodoxy, contrarianism and scientific curiosity, was the culture medium in which I matured.

My brother Harold was something of a philosopher and taught me the difference between inductive and deductive ways of thinking. The lesson that has always stayed with me was the proof of "Baum's theorem". Baum's theorem posits that all odd numbers are prime numbers and here is the proof. One is odd and prime, three is odd and prime, five is odd and prime, seven is odd and prime, nine is *experimental error*, eleven is odd and prime, thirteen is odd and prime…enough already, QED. In this way by the time I entered medical school on a State scholarship in 1955, the damage had been done yet at the same time my father had the wisdom to advise me not to make waves and draw attention to myself in case the Cossacks got to hear about it.

I qualified at Birmingham University in 1960 and became elected as a Fellow of the Royal College of Surgeons (FRCS) in 1965 following which I took some time out to embark on research into breast cancer. At that time there was no controversy regarding the treatment of the disease but I was determined to start one. In those days it was all so easy, all women were treated by radical mastectomy and if any of them died it was either the surgeons fault for not cutting away enough or the woman's fault for not presenting early enough. ("Experimental errors")

I then started reading avidly around this subject and soon learnt that there was only one man in the world who was making waves and seeing through this inductive farce, and that was Dr. Bernard (Bernie) Fisher in Pittsburgh PA. In the late 1960s Bernie was making himself enemies by taking on the whole of the surgical establishment and claiming they had got it wrong for the last 70 years. I was jealous that one man could make so many enemies and I wanted my share, so I took the initiative, abandoned my job at Kings College Hospital in 1970 and apprenticed myself to this great man and sure enough in no time at all I had enemies of my own.

I wasn't yet aware that I was suffering from *scepticaemia* and that didn't become apparent for another 9 or 10 years. In 1974, by which time I was an associate professor of surgery at the Welsh National School of Medicine in Cardiff, I was invited to address the World Cancer Congress in Florence on the controversy of radical mastectomy versus breast conserving surgery at the instigation of Bernie Fisher.

This was my first big break. I prepared a beautifully illustrated lecture and gave a barn storming performance and sure enough acquired even more enemies but, as I discovered later that week, I had also acquired some new friends who shared my point of view. Two days later on a beautiful balmy evening I was enjoying a quiet Campari orange in the Piazza della Signoria when 6 or 7 very friendly blond giants of Nordic extraction confronted me. They were mostly Swedish but one was from Norway and another from Denmark. They politely asked if they could join me and then bought the first of several rounds of drinks. The mood soon became boisterous and by the time I had retired to my hotel they had pledged allegiance to my iconoclastic cause. One week later the leader of this group, Karl Magnus Rudenstam, invited me to join a scientific steering committee for a new annual Nordic Oncology Course.

These courses turned out to be a great success partly because they took place on the ski slopes close to the Arctic Circle. In due course, as a reward for my work in educating young Nordic oncologists I was awarded an honorary doctorate in medicine at the University of Gothenburg. However education works both ways and in mid winter in 1987 I met a man who changed my life forever. He was born in Bohemia and came to Ireland as a refugee from Prague after the Russians occupied Czechoslovakia; he taught in the department of Community Health in Trinity College, Dublin and his name was Petr Skrabanek.

Shortly before his death from aggressive prostate cancer he published a book "The death of Humane Medicine and the rise of coercive healthism," that contained much of the material that he taught on the Nordic oncology course. Petr was a real scholar and was reluctant to waste time and risk life and limb sliding down a snow slope with wooden planks attached to his feet. I found Petr better company than the snow covered mountains so during the breaks for outdoor activities I chose to sit with him sipping schnapps and listening to him talk about the teachings of Michel de Montaigne, Voltaire and Sir Thomas Browne, two French and one English heretics, who through their iconoclastic writings, changed the history of the world and paved the way for the age of enlightenment.

Montaigne invented the literary term "essay" derived from the French word *essai,* meaning to put on trial. In his collection of essays he describes his life's work in testing his responses to different subjects and situations using his *ego* and *alter ego* as council for and against the case.

In one such essay he writes,

> "Why do doctors begin by practising on the credulity of their patients with so many false promises of a cure, if not to call the powers of the imagination to the aid of their fraudulent concoctions?" (Book 1, Chapter 21, "On the power of the imagination", 1580)

It is hard to believe that this was written over 400 years ago and here am I writing essays in the method invented by Montaigne whilst still addressing the same follies ascribed to 16th Century French citizens (See section on alternative medicine)

In 1764 Voltaire published his *Dictionnaire philosophique* in which he took the essay format one step further by organising them in alphabetical order and adding sardonic wit to better illuminate the follies and fallacies of that époque.

One of his aphorisms that resonates with me 250 years on, went something like this:

> "Faith consists in believing when it is beyond the power of reason to believe. It is not enough that a thing be possible for it to be believed".

The third in this unholy trinity, Sir Thomas Browne, is my favourite probably because he was English and wrote in the earthy, *in your face*, brand of the British Renaissance. I have three precious volumes of his collected works published in 1836. Thomas Browne was born in Cheapside in London in 1605 and went to study in at Pembroke College Oxford in 1623 as a "gentleman commoner". After taking a degree of MA he turned his studies to medicine. His first notable book was *Religio Medici* (The religion of a physician). He eventually settled in Norwich in East Anglia in 1636. For the rest of his long life he practised as a physician and spent his leisure writing essays. King Charles II knighted him in 1671. He died in 1682 at the age of 77. His son Edward Browne followed his father into the medical profession and ultimately was appointed as physician to King Charles II. As such, he was one of fourteen physicians who attended the deathbed of the monarch and contributed to the debauchery of quack remedies applied. [See box]

The Death of King Charles II

At eight o'clock on Monday morning February 2, 1685, Kings Charles II of England was being shaved in his bedroom. With a sudden cry he fell backwards and had a violent convulsion. Doctor Scarburgh, one of twelve or fourteen physicians called to treat the stricken King, recorded the efforts made to cure the patient.

As the first step in treatment the king was bled to the extent of a pint from a vein in his right arm. Next the shoulder was cut into and the incised area was "cupped" to suck out an additional eight ounces of blood. After this the drugging began. An emetic and purgative were administered. This was followed by an enema containing antimony, sacred bitters, rock salt, mallow leaves, violets, beetroot, camomile flower, fennel seed, linseed, cinnamon, cardamom seed, saphron, cochineal and aloes. The king's head was shaved and a blister raised on his scalp. A sneezing powder of hellebore root was administered and also a powder of cowslip flowers 'to strengthen the brain'.

The king's did not improve; indeed it grew worse and in the emergency forty drops of extract of human skull was administered to allay convulsions. A rallying dose of Raleigh's antidote was forced down the king's throat; finally bezoar stone was given.

'Alas after an ill –fated night his serene majesty's strength seemed exhausted to such a degree that the whole assembly of physicians lost hope and became despondent: still so as not to appear to fail in their duty in any detail, they brought into play the most active cordial.' As a sort of grand summary of the pharmaceutical debauch, a mixture of Raleigh's antidote, pearl julep, and ammonia was forced down the throat of the dying king.

Haggard's description of the treatment of King Charles from "Devils, Drugs and Doctors" (1929), Harper.

Many of Thomas Browne's essays were published posthumously, and like Montaigne, they were mostly written for his own pleasure. My three antiquarian books group these essays together in collections described as, *Religio Medici/Garden of Cyrus, Urn-Burial tracts etc.* and *Vulgar errors.* Like Montaigne and Voltaire, half of his output attempts to understand the follies of mankind and their capacity of making "vulgar errors" in observation and belief so that they are capable of ignoring reason in the name of faith. His other essays describe a bizarre collection of common beliefs that he dissects with the clear vision of an anatomist. There are hundreds to choose from but my two favourites are "*That a man hath one Rib less than a woman*" and "*That Jews stink*". Christian orthodoxy of the day taught a fundamentalist interpretation of the Bible. It therefore followed that if Eve were fashioned from Adam's rib, then Eve's descendents would always have one more rib than Adam's descendents. Browne doubted that and went to study anatomy in the Low Countries and made his business to count the number of ribs on both sides of the chest in male and female cadavers. This simple exercise in observational research refuted the religious belief but I suspect he kept quiet about that until close to his death. In book 4 of *"Vulgar errors"* chapter 10, I was shocked to learn that in 17th C *Merrie England* it was considered that you could always tell when a Jew was approaching by the stink that announced his presence. Browne does a beautiful hatchet job on this and although his language shares the convolutions and curlicues of the period you can hear the heavy irony when he explains why the theory has no rational basis and secondly that the empirical evidence adduced by sniffing in the proximity to a synagogue produces no different an odour than sniffing in proximity to a Church. He concludes that some individuals may stink but this unfortunate state is not generalizable to a specific race. For this I am much indebted to Sir Thomas and proud to continue in the steps of this great debunker of myths.

To return to Petr Skrabanek; in 1989 Petr along with his mentor in Dublin, professor James McCormick, published a book entitled "Follies and Fallacies in Medicine" continuing the tradition of the three giants of the age of enlightenment where, for the first time, the pathological state of *scepticaemia* is defined. (*Scepticaemia: An uncommon generalized disorder of low infectivity. Medical school education is likely to confer life-long immunity)

I give early warning: take care in reading any further as the bug might infect you.

Introduction

From the General to the Particular

In the same way that Thomas Browne structured his collection of essays from general principles to particular examples, I have structured this book from the general to the particular. Some people on meeting me for the first time and learning that I am a surgeon specializing in diseases of the breast, assume that my very narrow specialization would be accompanied by a narrowness of mind. I refute that misconception and claim that among my friends and colleagues who have become super specialists in their fields, I find those who are the most accomplished human beings are true renaissance men and women. For example I know one professor who is a leading authority on assisted fertilization and another a specialist in diseases of the upper gastro-intestinal tract, who sit in the House of Lords. They were not anointed as nobility because they knew a thing or two about IVF or Crohn's diseases. No, they were elevated to the upper chamber of our houses of parliament because of their wisdom and all round scholarship to advise governments of all political leanings, on matters concerning science, technology, ethics and humanitarianism. I cannot claim an accolade of such importance in the higher reaches of national governance but I hope that my breadth of knowledge has at least contributed to the education of several generations of medical students denying them the lifetime immunity to open-mindedness of conventional didactic teaching. I have therefore organized this book from the general to the particular in the following sections:

Scientific and Moral philosophy;
Medical Humanities;

Alternative medicine;
Cancer in general;
Breast cancer;
Screening for breast cancer;

And finally a section entitled "towards a synthesis", in which I attempt to describe an attitude of mind and code of conduct, which can incorporate the lessons of a lifetime in the practice of medicine with an open mind yet not so open as to let my brains slide out.

Scientific and Moral Philosophy

Chapter 1

Karl Popper Memorial Lecture

London School of Economics
November 2007
The Philosophical Surgeon:
In Defence of Evidence-Based Medicine

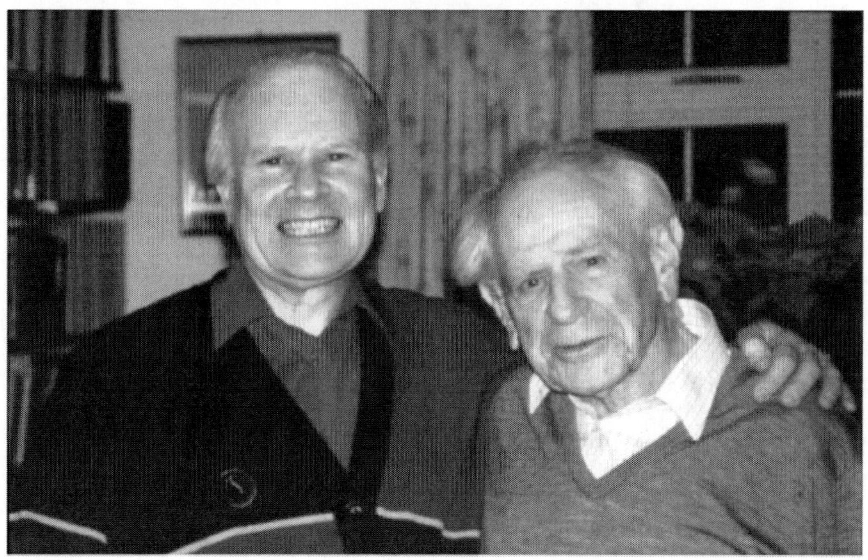

Sir Karl Popper and the author, 1992.

Introduction

I had always been interested in the history and philosophy of science since embarking on my academic career in the early 1970s. This was in part due to the influence of one of my brothers, Professor Harold Baum, who went on to become Dean of Life Science at Kings College, London. I even went so far as to list this interest, along with the history of fine art amongst the subjects I dabbled in, when composing my first entry into Who's Who. I identified myself as a Popperian for reasons of taxonomy and a wish to impress my friends. You can therefore imagine my surprised delight on hearing from my hero in person sometime in 1991, when I was invited to look after a close friend of Karl who had just been diagnosed with breast cancer. When I asked him "why me?" he replied that it was because of my entry in Who's Who.

If I wanted a surgeon to cut me open my first wish would be that he was a master of his craft, the fact that he might have an interest in philosophy would be well down on the list of personal traits I would be looking for.

Nevertheless things went well and I became pretty friendly with the old man in the last few years of his life. We exchanged letters on matters philosophical and I was invited to tea on the very day he took delivery of the first Russian translation of "The Open Society and its Enemies". In his excitement he signed a copy of the English version for me, which remains one of my most precious keepsakes. The last communication I had from Karl was a letter dated 4/1/93, referring to some papers I sent for him to critique upon which he commented favourably. The last line of his last letter read; "For me, the most interesting of your papers was, 'Limitations of non-science in Surgical Epistemology', I hope you may find time, one day, to discuss these issues with me." Sadly I didn't but that is the theme of my memorial lecture.

The Philosophical Surgeon

There is an old joke doing the rounds of the cocktail party circuit, which runs as follows: A hostess introduces two strangers to each other, one a doctor and the other a lawyer. The lawyer goes on to say 'Oh so you're a doctor. I must tell you this screamingly funny story about a surgeon'. To which the doctor replies 'I think before you go any further, I ought to warn you that I am a surgeon'. Quick as a flash the lawyer responds: 'in which case I will tell it very slowly!' Once again the stereotype of the surgeon is reinforced as an unthinking technician, so that the very title 'philosophical surgeon' might be read as an oxymoron.

In defence of the thinking surgeon, I wish to propose that a modern surgeon practicing evidence-based, humane and ethical medicine, must have a sound grounding in some of the fundamental principles of philosophy. I shall illustrate these principles, drawing on 40 years experience as a surgeon within the NHS and in particular my specialist practice in the diagnosis and management of breast cancer.

The Epistemology of Medicine

Epistemology is a bit of a mouthful that simply means the study or the theory of the growth of knowledge – or putting it another way, how is it that we know certain facts to be true. At the most simple level our observations can be misleading, and so called 'common sense' is no substitute for a systematic approach to the acquisition of knowledge. Primitive man 'knew' that the Earth was flat and that the Earth was the centre of the universe. For all intents and purposes it made little difference to the way of life in primitive communities, but these firmly held beliefs were false. The recognition that the world was round and that the universe was heliocentric rather than geocentric was a scientific observation of seismic importance in the history of mankind.

All undergraduates should understand this period of history where the theories of Copernicus and the observations of Galileo changed man's status in the universe, and opened minds to a systematic pursuit of knowledge from the age of enlightenment to the present day. The playwright Bertold Brecht put the following words into the mouth of Galileo: 'It is not the purpose of our science to open the gates to infinite wisdom but merely to set the limits to the extent of our ignorance.' If that is indeed the case for the study of cosmology, which has little impact on the day-to-day life of even the most sophisticated communities, how much more so does it apply to our lives when facing their premature end under the threat of cancer or cardiovascular disease.

Inductive Logic versus Deductive Logic

It was Aristotle and other great names of the golden age of Pericles in the ancient city of Athens, who were the first to apply a systematic approach to the pursuit of knowledge. They recognised that our conceptual model of the world around us was a figment of our imagination, and it was therefore necessary to systematically collect observations to challenge this view. These observations were built up into a conceptual model (hypothesis), and later observations were selected to corroborate this model.

The process of collecting observations in defence of a hypothesis is known as inductivism. Inductive logic was considered 'science' up until the eighteenth century, when the Scottish philosopher David Hume finally illustrated the poverty of the process. Perhaps the best way of illustrating the poverty of inductivism as it relates to our lives as medical practitioners is to consider the subject of *alternative medicine*.

When doctors attack alternative medicine or appear sceptical to its much-trumpeted claims, we are often accused of being bigots with closed minds, protecting a closed shop. Nothing could be further from the truth, but it has taken a layman, the late great John Diamond, to find the words to set the record straight. For that reason I would like to quote from his posthumously published book 'Snake Oil and other Preoccupations' [1].

> 'I am not an academic and this is not an academic book, even though the facts I list in it have a perfectly good scientific basis to them but when it comes to human motivation I am working blind. I can only guess why most people seem to prefer the unproven to the proven, the anecdotal to the rigorously demonstrated, and the so-called natural to the scientific'.

There is much within that passage, on the nature of proof, the nature of the scientific method, and the use and abuse of anecdotal evidence.

The alternative practitioner can trace his roots back to Galen in the second century, and a metaphysical belief system based on the balance of *natural humours*. For example, Galen believed that breast cancer was due to an excess of *black bile* (melancholia). Inductive support for this belief came from the observation that breast cancer was more common in post-menopausal women than pre-menopausal women, and this was thought to be because the menstrual flux in pre-menopausal women got rid of the putative excess of black bile. The therapeutic consequences of this belief therefore were purgation and venesection (bloodletting). The inductive 'proof' that this approach worked were the anecdotes about women with breast cancer who were treated by purgation and venesection, and who lived for several years after diagnosis. Those who died were the victims of the blood letter who didn't have the courage of his convictions, or the patient herself who lacked the constitutional vigour to sustain prolonged bloodletting.

There is a neo-Galenic doctrine, based on the view that breast cancer is indeed due to an imbalance of nature, only substituting *energy fields* for the natural humours. According to this view, to restore perfect health you have to restore the balance of these metaphysical *energy fields*. This might be achieved by acupuncture balancing out the yin and the yang, homeopathy (*simularis simulabum curantur),* or strange balancing diets. The Gerson diet in particular is very fashionable.

In fact, one of my patients, seeking to improve my education, gave me a book describing this approach [2]. The first half of the book formulates the hypothesis why this strange diet should improve the balance of the immune system, and the second half of the book consisted of 50 anecdotes of patients with cancer, who were only given six months to live by the medical profession, took the diet and lived for a long time.

The trouble with that kind of evidence is that although we know the numerator (50) we don't know the denominator – for example, 50 out of 1000 cases treated by neglect could indeed live for many years while the indolent disease progresses on the chest wall. Furthermore, from the evidence available in the book some of the diagnoses were a little bit shaky and the author neglects to mention whether or not these patients receive conventional treatment at the same time as the magic diet. Finally, I know of no oncologist who gives a patient six months to live. We may say that the median survival for a group with advanced cancer is six months, but among this group certain individuals may lie at extremes of survival. These individuals are the substance of the anecdote.

Perhaps I should leave the last word on this subject by quoting from Robert Park's wonderful book *Voodoo Science*. 'Alternative seems to define a culture rather than a field of medicine – a culture that is not scientifically demanding. It is a culture in which ancient accretions are given more weight than biological science and anecdotes are preferred over clinical trials. Alternative therapies steadfastly resist change often for centuries or even millennia, unaffected by scientific advances in the understanding of physiology or disease' [3]. If that is the case then who are the bigots and who are the ones with the closed minds?

Deductive Logic and the Randomised Controlled Trial

The alternative to alternative medicine, should be scientific medicine, not 'orthodoxy'. By science, I mean the application of deductive logic. The deductive approach starts with the formulation of the hypothesis, but for a start the hypothesis must be rational in its explanation of the disease process or therapeutic intervention. By 'rational' I mean built upon the growth of knowledge of human biology and physiology from the past 100 years or so, without invoking magic or metaphysical principles.

Even so, the new hypothesis is still perceived as a fictional account of reality and subjected to rigorous test by the design of experiments challenging the new theory with the 'hazard of refutation'. These experiments in medical or surgical therapeutics must have control groups treated by observation, placebo or 'best available therapy'. Without the control group we merely have a series of anecdotal reports. What I have just described is in fact a randomised controlled trial.

Breast Cancer and the Randomised Controlled Trial

As I have mentioned, up until the eighteenth century, if breast cancer was treated at all, was treated according to the principles of Galen. It wasn't until the mid-nineteenth century that it became widely accepted that cancer was a disease of cellular pathology originating within the breast and spreading centrifugally along the lymphatic system. The therapeutic consequence of this belief led surgeons to embark on radical surgery that involved removing the breast and all the regional lymphatics. It was left to William Halsted in the 1890s to refine the operation into the classic radical mastectomy, with the intention of ridding the body of the primary cancer and its lymph node secondaries. Sadly, the only support for this radical treatment was anecdotal. If the patient survived it was due to the success of the surgeon. If the patient died it was either because the patient came too late or the surgeon lacked the courage of his convictions to complete a truly radical operation.

It was only when Dr Bernard Fisher in the 1960s challenged the conceptual model of the disease that progress started to be made. In other words an antithesis was constructed to challenge the prevailing dogma. Fisher taught that contrary to popular belief, breast cancer cells spread throughout the body through the venous drainage of the breast, and at the time of clinical presentation of the disease, the majority of breast cancers were in fact systemic disorders. If that was indeed the case then there are two therapeutic consequences. Firstly, that radical surgery is shutting the stable door after the horse has bolted. Therefore the role of local therapy is local control, which would equally well be achieved by breast conserving techniques such as lumpectomy and radiotherapy. The second therapeutic corollary is that if indeed the disease is systemic at the time of diagnosis then the only way to improve cure rates is through chemotherapy or hormone therapy.

However, the greatness of Dr Fisher, ably supported by surgical acolytes all around the world, was not simply to accept a new set of beliefs in place of an old set of beliefs, but to challenge the new paradigm using deductive logic: in other words, through randomised controlled trials. One of the great success stories of modern medicine has been the painstaking series of randomised controlled trials in the management of early breast cancer over the past 30 years. We now know with extreme confidence that breast conservation is a safe alternative to radical mastectomy, although not in itself improving cure rates, greatly enhancing the patient's quality of life. We also know with extreme confidence that treatment using either endocrine or cytotoxic regimens will improve survival. The final demonstration of that truth has been the dramatic fall in breast cancer mortality in the UK and North America since 1985, following the first publication of the world overview of trials [4].

Using breast cancer as an example, we can demonstrate that the philosophy of science that underpins the randomised controlled trials has led to the dramatic improvement in length of life and quality of life for women inflicted with this dread disease. However this isn't the end of the story, as new biological hypotheses are being generated with new therapeutic consequences, all of which will be tested in the randomised controlled trial, which is now accepted as the most scientific and ethical way of conducting medicine in times of uncertainty.

Conclusion

Karl Popper inspired me, taught me to think critically and changed my life from that of a technocrat to that of a scientist. Science fed my curiosity and my original observations provided an open ticket to travel the world. I shall therefore leave the last word to him;

> "It is not truisms that science unveils. Rather, it is part of the greatness and the beauty of science that we can learn, through our own critical investigations, that the world is utterly different from what we ever imagined-"

References

[1] *Snake Oil and other Preoccupations*, John Diamond, Vintage Random House UK, 2001

[2] *A Cancer Therapy: results of fifty cases and the cure of advanced cancer by diet therapy*, Max Gerson, Gerson Institute Bonita, California, 1986.

[3] *Voodoo Science*, Robert Park, Oxford University Press, Oxford, 2000.

[4] 'Sudden fall in breast cancer death rates in England & Wales', Beral V, Hermon C, Reeves G, Peto R,. *Lancet* 1995; 345:1642-3.

Chapter 2

Plato's Socratic Dialogues and the Epistemology of Modern Medicine

Journal of the Royal Society of Medicine: 2010 Dec;103(12):484-9

James May[1], Michael Baum[2] and Susan Bewley[3]

[1]General Practitioner, Lambeth Walk Group Practice, London

[2]Professor Emeritus of Surgery, University College London, Director clinical trials group; Royal Free and UCL Medical School, Centre for Clinical Science

[3]Consultant Obstetrician, Kings Health Partners, c/o Women's Services, St Thomas' Hospital, Westminster Bridge Rd, London

Plato's recordings of the dialogues of Socrates, the greatest thinker of ancient Greece, are precious items in Western philosophy, culture and science. Socratic method still informs our teaching; wise medical instructors do not fill students' heads with "facts" but adopt a feigned position of ignorance from which to ask probing questions so they arrive eventually at insights that are the true pre-requisite for gaining knowledge. Furthermore, these dialogues represent the birth of scientific method; starting with the recognition of one's ignorance we learn that posing pertinent questions is halfway to solving them.

In the dialogue known as "apology" (*apologia* - speaking in defence of one's beliefs and actions), Socrates is at his cunning best. Holding a cup of deadly hemlock, Meletus, one of his Interlocutors, charges Socrates with atheism and scientific sophistry because his curiosity leads him to make enquiries into the earth and sky.

In his defence, Socrates describes how Chaerephon consulted the oracle of Delphi who confirmed that Socrates was the wisest of all men. This was a paradox to be resolved as Socrates considered himself an ignorant man. Perhaps the oracle sent Chaerephon on a divine mission to see how an ignorant man could be wiser than politicians, poets, prophets and seers? Ultimately Socrates traps Meletus into agreeing that the ignorant man who starts from the premise of knowing little is the wisest of all, thus demonstrating that posing the right questions is the secret of epistemology in all walks of life. Despite winning the argument, Socrates still had to take the hemlock.

We present a true sequence of e-mails exchanged between three clinicians contemplating the epistemology of modern medicine. Instead of sitting in the shade of an oak tree our discourse took place though the WorldWideWeb.

Retrospectively, the thought sequences had an eerie similarity to 'apology' suggesting inspiration from Ancient Greek ghosts of Socrates (JM) and Meletus (MB) overseen by Athena (SB), Goddess of Wisdom. References and clarifications were added later.

****

Socrates: Is Empiricism [an assertion that knowledge arises from sense experience] a way of life in the search for knowledge in the practice of medicine, or merely one useful tool among many? Are RCTs [randomised controlled trials] the only way of doing trials? Could a Bayesian approach be used sometimes? [1] Bookies don't start from the assumption that all horses are equal. They calculate on a system that collates the horse's overall form with how it did in its last race. Therefore why should we, when comparing treatments, assume at the outset that all are equal?

Meletus: I don't trust Bayesian maths. This is based on prior belief systems and these are often evidence-free or even based on prejudice. I would challenge anyone to show me one example where the Bayesian approach predicted a reliable outcome to clinical research. This is different to the observation that when a medical condition has a predictable natural history then a treatment with spectacular results needs no RCT. e.g. penicillin, appendicectomy.

Athena: Have I missed something? How can Bayesian maths not be trusted? It's just maths. Is it the uses people claim for it rather than the thing itself that is problematic? My understanding was that all medical diagnosis is based on Bayesian logic. The Wizard and the Gatekeeper article helps understand this [2]: there is a prior probability that your next patient with abdominal pain has appendicitis; this is different if you are a GP or a hospital surgeon after primary care filter; thus every question you ask or physical sign you elicit or even the GPs "test of time" – i.e. review in a day or next week - should add to the accuracy of the posterior probability, as per Socrates' analogy of the bookie. Diagnosis shouldn't be based on prior 'belief' but prior observations.

There has been a Bayesian RCT - the Growth Restriction Intervention Trial, based on obstetricians' prior beliefs/clinical wisdom whether growth restricted fetuses would be better off delivered prematurely or left in utero. It worked on individual equipoise without set criteria with a combined short (death) and long-term (disability) outcome. The stillbirth and death before hospital discharge rates were equal, despite a 4 day difference of gestation, but caesareans were less frequent when waiting conservatively. Handicap was higher in <31 week group if delivered immediately. The trial was criticised (of course). You might be right that it still leaves clinicians open to their prejudices but it was quite a milestone between Bayesians and Frequentists[1]. It provided evidence that babies should be left in utero, if possible.

Meletus: It's not just maths, it's value laden maths with values weighted according to prior beliefs or "experience". That might work reasonably with diagnosis - although one wag once put it that experience implied making the same mistakes again. When it comes to treatment of conditions with an unknown or unpredictable natural history then as far as I'm concerned Bayesian approaches are simply inductive logic, selecting the evidence that reinforces your prejudices. If we had used a Bayesian approach instead of the deductive approach of RCTs we would still be doing radical mastectomy as the prior belief was set so far away to the left of the null hypothesis that no amount of data could shift it into the non-inferiority domain of breast conservation surgery. [3]

Socrates: But once we have RCT results, don't we have to use inductive logic if we are to apply them in practice? There must be a degree of generalization from the particular result. Or should we only believe a drug is effective if our patient was involved in the RCT? Does medicine in practice

[1] Frequentism: a statistical perspective that focuses on the frequency with which an observed value is expected in numerous trials in an effort to avoid anything savouring of matters of opinion.

cease to be scientific because it uses such induction? Am I misunderstanding what you mean by induction?

Meletus: I attach my Karl Popper memorial lecture in my defence! [4]

[After a pause]

Socrates: I would like to respond to your excellent lecture: by distinguishing between 'Inductivism' (an entire view of scientific methodology) which I agree is thoroughly discredited, and 'induction' itself, which is *"any inference where the claim made by the conclusion goes beyond the claim jointly made by the premises"* [5] . If we throw out induction with 'Inductivism' we lose something we all use daily in medical practice (I will argue). Hume explained this very clearly. Induction, in his argument, uses an empirical experience (a past event by definition) as the foundation to predict future events. He says there is no empirical foundation for doing this. He acknowledges that we all do it. He does it. But there is no foundation for it.

"It is impossible, therefore, that any arguments from experience can prove this resemblance of the past to the future, since all these arguments are found on the supposition of that resemblance. Let the course of things be allowed hitherto ever so regular, that alone, without some new argument or inference, proves not that for the future it will continue so. In vain do you pretend to have learned the nature of bodies from your past experience. Their secret nature, and consequently all their effects and influence, may change without any change in their sensible qualities. This happens sometimes, and with regard to some objects. Why may it not happen always, and with regard to all objects? What logic, what process of argument secures you against this supposition? My practice, you say, refutes my doubts. But you mistake the purport of my question. As an agent, I am quite satisfied in the point; but as a philosopher who has some share of curiosity, I will not say scepticism, I want to learn the foundation of this inference."

Athena: And how does this relate to modern medical practice?

Socrates: Applying RCT evidence to the patient in front of me is exactly this sort of inductive move Hume says is not justified on the basis of empirical knowledge. This is the classic problem of induction (as I understand it). Inductive inferences assume what has been called the 'uniformity of nature': that the future will resemble the past. This is a fundamental philosophical assumption of science. The future is not based on empirical observation – by definition!

I have put all this together in a logical form.

Consider the following deductive arguments:

1. a. Using past evidence to predict future events is an inductive process.
   b. Medical practice uses RCT observations and applies them to patients in the present/future
   c. Conclusion: Medical practice is based on induction
2. a. Inductive logic is unscientific
   b. Medical practice is based on induction
   c. Conclusion: Medical practice is unscientific

Because they are deductive arguments, in order to disagree with the conclusions you would have to disagree with one or other of the premises (assuming I have framed the arguments correctly).....

I would disagree with the premise 2.a. - that Inductive logic is unscientific. What would you say?

Meletus: A good challenge. I think frequentists in clinical methodology accept this argument in part and have been trying to address it for some time indirectly through power calculations. Strictly, it is true that the result of an RCT applies only to the population studied. The more prescriptive the entry criteria the more difficult it is to generalize beyond the trial population.

Because of this I belong to the pragmatic wing of the EBM [evidence-based medicine] movement. We believe that the larger the sample size and the broader the entry criteria and the intention to treat analysis the more unlikely it becomes that the result can't be applied to the patient in front of you....

Athena: Too many double negatives!

Meletus: ...It becomes statistically improbable that your patient will respond in a different way - that is beyond the 95% confidence interval of the trial result. Furthermore, if there are such outliers we are duty bound to explain them. In other words, if there is a defined sub-group who demonstrate statistical heterogeneity from the main group, we can learn from them. I've described this as "biological fall-out". The larger the sample size, the more we can look at outliers and the more we can learn about the disease and its treatment. That is why large collaborative groups try to collect tens of thousands of patients or carry out meta-analysis, not out of megalomania, nor just to find tiny incremental improvements for the whole group, but ultimately to personalize care. Eventually this allows the patient and doctor to make their own knowledge-based informed choice. It's a little better than "ignorance-based medicine".

Socrates: A fine clinician's answer with good research backing, which is pragmatic and sensible and something to aspire to. But it does not avoid the charge of induction. It is simply an inductive argument, which attempts to increase the support of the truth of the conclusion to a higher degree, but does not and cannot guarantee the truth of the conclusion. The conclusion is not a deductive conclusion flowing inescapably from the premises.

Popper, I think, would say that the only amount of powering that gives empirical justification is infinite powering. Anything less is finite, and a finite number is always infinitely small compared to infinity. So, the problem of induction remains because there is no certain "medical proof" based on experience. I agree with every word you say, as long as you admit it is a process of induction!

Meletus: My dictionary has nine meanings for induction so we are in danger of generating a futile semantic exercise. By chance, 'inductile' ("not pliable; unyielding to influences") appears above 'induction', a word I've never used but appears apposite. [6] I suggest that RCTs are exercises in the method of the hypothetico-deductive cascade that is the never-ending, constantly refined approximation to an objective reality. The treatments that are the therapeutic consequences of the biological model that best represents our transient approximation to reality are therefore the best available at the time. Our practice, however, is NOT "inductile" as it will yield to treatments that emerge as we improve our approximation to a truth that is always beyond the reach of us mere mortals.

Socrates: I hope you agree it's worth putting the discussion in some context. It is interesting that our views will seem to converge almost completely by the end. I agree definitions are complicated. I was, however, trying to use what I understand to be the mainstream philosophical meaning of induction: 'any inference where the claim made by the conclusion goes beyond the claim jointly made by the premises.' You might be interested in a quote from Popper which relates to our discussion about powering; *"One (could) ascribe to the hypothesis a certain probability... on the basis of an estimate of the ratio of all tests passed by it to all the tests which have not yet been attempted ... This estimate can, as it happens, be computed with precision, and the result is always that the probability is zero"* [7]

In other words, no amount of positive empirical data can ever raise the probability of a scientific theory above zero., Now is the time to question if you are a thorough going Popperian! On the basis of experience alone, however, it would seem that Popper is right (as most philosophers accept) – there is no purely empirical foundation for scientific theories.

Meletus: The problem is clear.

Socrates: If we step back, we can see why this is worth discussing. The questions seem to be "Is there such a thing as a systematic approach to knowledge that distinguishes science from pseudo-science? If there is, what is it? If there isn't, is there anything useful that can be said to make a distinction?"

Popper's rejection of induction is part of the problem – not part of the solution I think. Popper successfully critiques the verification principle of logical positivism. Using empirical data and logic alone we cannot 'verify' a scientific theory. He thus rejects induction, rejects verification and opts for falsification (whereby a true scientific theory is indentified as one which is falsifiable in principle).

If we follow the skepticism (or curiosity) of Hume and Popper, then we have to conclude that we cannot find firm foundations in science based on empirical justification alone.

Athena: What about actual scientists?

Socrates: For these reasons I am not a Popperian (is that heresy?), and neither are most practicing scientists, whilst agreeing that modern science still rests on his insights as much as any other individual. Since Popper - and probably because of Popper's 'anti-foundationalist' insights - many philosophers of science have given up on a 'systematic approach to knowledge'. Practicing scientists do seem convinced to a high degree of the truth of a particular theory, which is more than Popper seems to allow for. There is no *singular* scientific method, whether logical positivism or falsification. There are instead a variety of methods used in different degrees in different contexts.

Meletus: But surely we are left without either being able to define 'true science' or to identify and reject 'pseudo-science'? Homeopaths will always be able to claim, as some do, that RCTs are not the appropriate tool for investigating homeopathy.

Socrates: It is, I concede, more challenging for those of us wishing to promote public understanding of science-based medicine. This culture is philosophically justified in being skeptical of statements regarding science which speak in terms of 'facts', 'proofs' and 'certainties'. Popper has successfully refuted this approach to science.

Scientific epistemology is complex. Whilst the place of empiricism is perhaps weaker than we might like, it would be a mistake to try to find 'certainty' somewhere else. Empirical observation remains essential, not merely important, for good science. Philosophically speaking it is a *necessary* part of science, but it is not *sufficient* for good science. There will always be assumptions (such as the uniformity of nature) which themselves are not empirically verifiable but which we need to make in order to do good science.

Athena: I feel a bit weak....

Socrates: Don't. One response I favour is called 'Critical Realism'. There is a *real* world out there, real things can be known about it, and we need to be highly *critical* in our epistemology, always accepting that we might be wrong, but also believing that it is possible to be right (just not with certainty). What critical realism looks like in detail will vary from discipline to discipline. Rather than signing up to a particular scientific method as 'the right way', this is described as a humble epistemology. Far from giving license to justify pseudo-science, critical realists constantly work to submit knowledge claims to a higher authority than personal whims and prejudices – reality itself.

To 'understand' is literally to 'stand under'. Too often in history people have seen 'knowledge' as a conquest of reality rather than a submission to it. Instead of recognizing true science by possession of correct methodology, it might be better to identify a moral element; the virtue of humility. By this standard 'pseudo-science' is best identified as arrogantly failing to submit 'knowledge' claims to reality.

I therefore think that the aims of HealthWatch* would be best achieved with a gentle and humble confidence rather than speaking of certainties. [9]

I realize that scientists who are generally more 'modernist' by temperament find this approach a little namby-pamby. However, I think tentative statements are actually more persuasive than absolutist statements – we can leave such 'certainties' to the hucksters and fraudsters, whilst being confident that they are wrong. This seems to me to be exactly what you expressed much more concisely than me in an earlier email. A "cascade that is the never ending, constantly refined approximation to an objective reality" – but please consider that it may not be as Popperian as it first appears, and the "hypothetico-deductive cascade" is not the only game in town.

Meletus: I declare that I am no longer a Popperian but a Critical Realist. Philosophers have the advantage over clinicians that their *belle penses* cannot kill people first hand although, as Popper prophesied, [10] extreme ideologies from the left and the right will kill millions. Nevertheless we clinicians have to make decisions on a daily basis in the face of uncertainty and learn from our

* [1]Our only worry is that around the time of this interchange JM (Socrates) was elected chairman of the UK charity Healthwatch that may yet prove to be his poisoned chalice!

mistakes. This is an exercise in humility whereas "experience" (in the sense of 'the way things have always been done') simply repeats past mistakes. As you describe so eloquently, a good clinician must have many qualities above and beyond technical skills. Amongst these are humility, scepticism and a willingness to subject favoured ideas to the hazard of refutation. It seems that we have closed the gap between our starting positions.

Athena: Gentlemen, it appears that Socrates has won the argument. I wonder if we should share what we have learned: that we must hold our medical knowledge lightly and with humility, with confidence rather than certainty, and that we need constantly to be asking questions of our preferred epistemological theories?

****

Conflicts of interest: None declared.

References

[1] Benson Hugh H. 2000, Socratic Wisdom: The Model of Knowledge in Plato's Early Dialogues, New York: Oxford University Press.

[2] Mathers N. and Hodgkin P. *The Gatekeeper and the Wizard: a fairy tale.* BMJ 1989;298(6667): 172-4.

[3] GRIT Study Group. A randomised trial of timed delivery for the compromised preterm fetus: short term outcomes and Bayesian interpretation. *BJOG.* 2003 Jan;110(1):27-32.

[4] Fisher B, Jeong J-H, Anderson S, Bryant J, Fisher ER, Wolmark N. Twenty five-year follow-up of a randomized trial comparing radical mastectomy, total mastectomy,and total mastectomy followed by irradiation. *N Engl J Med* 2002;347:567-75.

[5] Baum M. Karl Popper Memorial. Lecture; LSE November 2007. The philosophical surgeon: in defence of evidence- based medicine. www2.lse.ac.uk/PublicEvents/pdf/20071106_Popper.pdf

[6] Definition of 'Induction', Cambridge Dictionary of Philosophy, 2nd Edition, General Editor Robert Audi, Cambridge, 1999.

[7] David Hume. An Inquiry Concerning Human Understanding (1748; Indianapolis: Bobbs-Merrill, 1965), pp. 51-52 (section 4.2 in the original)

[8] Popper KR; *The Logic of Scientific Discovery*, Routledge Classics, 2002, p255.
[9] May J. http://www.healthwatch-uk.org/newsletterarchive/nlett67.pdf p4.
[10] Popper KR. *The open society and its enemies,* volume 2. Hegel & Marx, Routledge, London, 1992.

Chapter 3

Justice

"Fiat justitia ruat coelum"
Let there be justice or the heavens fall

On September 11th 2001 the heavens did appear to fall in New York. A bunch of terrorists fuelled by an insane vision of injustice in the world and with total disrespect for the value of life, flew human bombs into the World Trade centre. Whilst not condoning for a minute their obscene notion of justice, consider for a moment these two items from the British Medical Journal, January 26th 2002.

"We all have AIDS"

"In occupied nations during World War II, the Nazis ordered Jews to wear a yellow star. The Danish King, Christian X threatened that, if Danish Jews were to wear the yellow star, he would too. If some Danes were under siege, then all Danes were under siege. Now we all have AIDS. In Botswana 36% of adults are infected with HIV---

Three million human beings died of AIDS in the year 2000, 2.4 million of them in sub Saharan Africa"

This very moving article then goes on to explain that these nations cannot afford the preventive or therapeutic measures to defeat this modern black death and the West stands idly by. [1]

US "boutique medicine" could threaten care for the majority.

"In return for a yearly membership fee of $1,500 the doctors contract to provide patients with annual physical examinations, same day appointments, 24 hour doctor availability, co-coordinated referrals to specialists and a promise to limit the practice to 600 patients (*per doctor)*". [2]

What this truly demonstrates is that half the world are dying prematurely for want of resources whilst the other half is exposed to "disease mongering" with annual check ups to keep the oversupply of doctors gainfully employed!

That should engender a sense of righteous indignation unless your conscience is truly atrophied.

What is justice?

The homily in the introduction illustrates the fact that it is easier to recognize injustice when you see it than to define justice in abstract terms.

The shorter Oxford English dictionary defines justice as-"The quality of being (morally) just or righteous"

Lord Chief Justice Devlin provided a more useful definition-"We can use the word to mean social justice and then we say that the law is just if it conforms to some social principle, such that all men are equal; that is justice *in rem.*"[3]

Note the distinction between the law and justice.

However as far as the practice of medicine is concerned Tom Beauchamp makes it clear that our primary concern is distributive justice; (BMJ 26/01/2002.)

"The principle of justice is really many principles about the distribution of benefits and burdens- to cite one example, an egalitarian theory of justice implies that if there is a departure from equality of distribution of health care benefit and burdens, such a departure must serve the common good and enhance the position of those who are least advantaged in society."[4]

That definition adheres to the philosophical school of "utilitarianism" first given voice by Jeremy Bentham the founder of my university. To paraphrase Bentham: the creation of happiness is the main goal in life and all our actions must be for the greatest good for the greatest number. The danger of this approach of course is uncontrolled search for a Utopia, which foundered at the Berlin wall.

It can therefore be judged that the principle of justice will often be in conflict with the principle of autonomy. In fact most of the toughest ethical dilemmas we face result from the quite appropriate tension between the ethical principles of justice and autonomy.

The parable of the starfish:

My late brother, Professor David Baum, was a paediatrician of great distinction who died in office as President of the Royal College of Paediatrics and Child Health. He had a massive myocardial infarction whilst leading a charity bike ride to raise money for the children in the camps of Kosovo. He was committed to equality of global health care for children in the name of justice. He was fond of quoting the parable of the starfish.

An old man walking the beach at dawn noticed a boy picking up a starfish and throwing it into the sea. When asked why the boy explained that the stranded starfish would die if left to lie in the morning sun. "But there are millions of starfish on the beach". Said the old man. "How can you efforts make a difference?" The boy picked up another starfish." It makes a difference to this one," he said.

One can sympathize with the old man when faced with the enormity of the task and also with boy whose action saves one life. As surgeons we have the dual responsibility to care for the individual and to oversee the just distribution of scarce resources in our clinics, our hospital, our health district, our nation and the under-privileged of the third world. I anticipate your cry; "We are practical men Professor how on earth are we to achieve these goals". For a start whenever we are prioritizing our waiting lists we are exercising the principle of justice. We must resist the politician's waiting list initiatives and insist clinical need comes before political expediency. In the inevitable wrangle over hospital resources always remember your freedom to carry out as many varicose veins as you damn well like may mean another old lady waits another year for a hip replacement. At a national level remember that the £40,000,000 (It's shot up to £100M since I wrote this) spent annually on mammographic screening might allow more humane living conditions in the psycho-geriatric ward. Also remember our global responsibility-"we all have AIDS". The best way we can discharge this responsibility as surgeons is to encourage and reward our senior residents for taking leave of absence to work in the third world. This will increase the number of doctors in the host country and provide better experience than a 40-hour week in a teaching hospital! Finally as a consultant –take a sabbatical and save some starfish from the sun. I know many who have done so and the reward is in the smiles of those who have lived life without hope or expectation of reaching adulthood.

References

[1] Berwick D. "We all have AIDS": case for reducing the cost of HIV drugs to zero. *BMJ* 324; 214-216: 2002.

[2] News ; *BMJ* 324;187: 2002.

[3] The Judge, Patrick Devlin, Oxford University Press , Oxford 1981

[4] Beauchamp TL., *The four- principles approach.* In; Principles of health care ethics, Editor Raanan Gillon, John Wiley and Sons, Chichester.New York. Brisbane. Toronto, Singapore. 1994 pp 3-12.

Chapter 4

The Roles of the Learned Societies in Improving Quality of Life in the Context of Globalization

Bangkok, Thailand 2011
Cancer care and Quality of Life
(Annals of Medicine and Surgery
Volume 1, Complete, Pages 16-18, 2012)

Thou shalt love thy neighbour as thyself. Leviticus 19:18

I am deeply honoured to have been asked to contribute to this historic occasion when learned societies from Thailand, France, Germany, Australia, New Zealand, the USA, India, Bangladesh, China and the United Kingdom, gather together to consider the problems facing the world in the context of the new challenges thrown up by Globalization. Out of respect for this occasion and by way of introduction, I would like to indulge myself with a short philosophical discourse.

I therefore choose to start my presentation by recalling the Old Testament commandment shown above, to remind us all that whatever race, religion or culture we come from, the simple command to love ones neighbour as ourselves, is the bedrock of civilization. In response to this command we have to ask ourselves two simple questions, a) how do we best express our love? And b) who do we consider to be our neighbour?

If one loves oneself then what is your single most important gift you would grant yourself? Ask anyone this question and they most always reply, the gift of good health. Therefore if you love others then the gift you want for them is also good health. These others who you should love in an unconditional way are your parents, your spouse, your children and grandchildren. I have 9 of the last category and these are the easiest to love unconditionally. I might then go on to joke that I hate my neighbours, that that is of course taking the words of the bible too literally. To whom does this duty or commandment to love extend. How wide is this circle of love? : The immediate family, the extended family, our village, our tribe or our Nation state? The answer to this is simple and contained within the very title of this symposium. With globalisation of commerce, social network information technology and relative ease of travel, the concept of the global village has matured and with this the duty of care from those countries that are resource rich to those countries that are resource poor, becomes an ethical imperative.

In summary therefore if we love our neighbour as ourselves, then we cannot stand by and watch them suffer nor must we squander scarce resources for tiny incremental improvements in health care for the rich whilst the poor of this world die prematurely from easily preventable or treatable disease. However, to put these high minded ambitions into practice on a grand scale is beyond the wit of one simple surgeon but I can at least illustrate the principles involved using the example of one disease that is responsible for the premature deaths of thousands of women round the world every day of the week; and that is carcinoma of the breast.

Outcome Measures

There are only two meaningful outcome measures in the evaluation of health care. Simply put; they are length of life (LOL) and quality of life (QOL). All other outcomes are surrogate and however compelling the results of screening, blood tests and medical images might be, they may not translate into improvements in LOL and QOL. [1] This is never truer than in the discussion of cancer care. LOL is of course easy to measure but even cancer "survival" statistics can be misleading unless they translate into mortality reduction ("Survival" meaning LOL from point of diagnosis, whilst mortality counts the number of age matched individuals dying from the disease on a year by year basis. Merely frame shifting the point of diagnosis “to the left” can artefactually extend survival without affecting mortality if the patient still dies at a predetermined point). QOL is not that easy to measure, but psychometric instruments for this purpose have been available since the mid 1970s and are constantly refined and validated. [2,3]

I will now illustrate these important generic issues by discussing breast cancer prevention, screening, surgery, systemic therapy and radiotherapy. The intention is to concentrate on real advances that are transferable to resource poor parts of the world whilst learning from the extravagant errors made by some of the wealthiest nations of the world, who have demonstrated that wealth and wisdom don’t always go hand in hand. I will end with a discussion about a new radiotherapy technique that is a perfect exemplar of transferable appropriate technology that happened earlier this year between my own department at University College London and Professor Kris Chatamara’s department at the Queen Sirikit breast cancer centre here in Bangkok.

Prevention

It is an old cliché that prevention is better than cure. As the incidence of breast cancer shows an almost linear correlation with the GDP of nations then maybe the resource rich nations of the world have something to learn from the resource poor. Of course that is a gross over simplification because cancers of most types increase in incidence with age and expectation of life is directly correlated with the wealth of nations. However if one recalculates these numbers with adjustment for age, the resource poor sections of the globe have a lower incidence of the disease. The best advice therefore, for resource poor parts of the world, is not to ape the lifestyle choices of the women living in northern Europe or North America. [4]

Screening

We have now reached a point where the majority of women in the resource rich parts of the world are breast cancer aware and present with disease that has the potential for cure. It is likely that this in part might have contributed to the welcome fall in mortality we have experienced over the last

20 years. [5] Breast cancer "awareness" is not high technology but dependant of public health education and resources focused on this alone are likely to generate greater dividends than screening of any kind. If the resource poor nations of the world are to learn anything from our mistakes of the past, then they need to recognize the folly of the widespread adoption of mammographic screening in Europe and North America. Screening has "a great future behind it"!

Screening illustrates all of the crimes described in my introduction, reliance on surrogate endpoints and the injustice of squandering scarce resources on interventions of trivial incremental gain, whilst the rest of the world can go to hell. "Catch it early" is the mantra and "save a life and save a breast" is the refrain. "Catch it early" means detecting the cancer at a pre-clinical stage. That is a surrogate end point that fails to translate into improving LOL and QOL. Screening does NOT save lives and paradoxically increases the mastectomy rates in screened populations. It is not the purpose of this paper to indulge in a diatribe against screening, as I have much of positive value to describe, furthermore to explain in detail why so many experts round the world have reached this position, would occupy almost all the time and space made available to me, instead I draw your attention to a rich bibliography of recent publications that support my contention. [5, 6, 7, 8, 9, 10, 11]

Surgery

In the 1960s radical mastectomy was the treatment of choice and "pathological clearance" was used as the surrogate marker for success. Yet the patients continued to die of metastatic disease in spite of "clear margins".

A revolutionary conceptual model of the disease was elaborated in the 1970s that led to a change of therapeutic approaches. [12] Instead of looking at the disease as an anatomical challenge that might be cured by surgery alone, it was considered a biological challenge with outcomes predetermined on the extent of occult metastatic disease present at the time of diagnosis. This then lead on to a series of trials with breast conserving surgery as a challenge to radical mastectomy with the objective of improving QOL. After decades of fierce debate and clinical trials we have now reached a consensus that breast conserving surgery (BCS) whenever technically feasible should be the default treatment. [13] That should be good news for resource poor nations because

BCS is quicker and requires fewer days of hospitalization than a mastectomy with our without reconstruction, but with two important caveats.

Firstly, the onus is on the woman herself to present when her tumour is small enough for BCS and as stated above, that is dependent on public health education.

Secondly BCS is only a safe alternative if accompanied by 3 to 6 weeks of radical radiotherapy that is a labour intense and high technology intervention. That also implies that the patient has easy access to a radiotherapy centre. I will deal with the solution to this problem at the end of this paper.

Adjuvant Systemic Therapy

BCS plus radiotherapy may indeed be non-inferior to radical mastectomy and thus improve QOL, but that alone does not improve LOL. To deal with that problem we need to look elsewhere. The paradigm shift in our contemporary understanding of breast cancer, posited the concept that the disease had to be considered a systemic disorder at the point of diagnosis [12] Should that be the case then to improve LOL some form of adjuvant systemic therapy (AST) must be indicated. Randomised controlled trials of AST using chemotherapeutic regimens and endocrine agents, started in the mid 1970s and constantly refined to this day, have confirmed their potential to improve LOL. The 30-40% reduction in breast cancer mortality we've enjoyed in Europe since the mid 1980s has recently been attributed to the introduction of AST with no contribution from screening, using the WHO database. [6] Complex chemotherapy regimens are costly and difficult to deliver; yet tamoxifen, a drug that has been credited with 60% of the improvement in breast cancer mortality [14], is now available as a cheap generic compound.

Unfortunately endocrine agents such as tamoxifen, are only of value in oestrogen receptor positive [ER+] cases, so the onus is on the resource rich parts of the world to develop less costly and less complex chemotherapy regimens for the developing parts of the world rather than squandering more and more of their GDP on miniscule incremental improvements that offer at best a few more months of "progression free survival", another bogus surrogate for LOL as exemplified by the recent scandal with Avastin. [15]

Radiotherapy

I would like to begin this section with an anecdote. I frequently look after patients with breast cancer from the UAE. They come to London for diagnostic work up and surgery and return home for postoperative radiotherapy and AST. One woman, who lives in Dubai, had to make the daily trek by car, one and a half hours each way, to Al-Ain for her radiotherapy. This involved 42 return journeys. On one occasion her driver fell asleep and they were involved in a serious crash. The injuries she received have to be considered as serious adverse events related to post operative radiotherapy. It is of course a pity that a wealthy city like Dubai with over two million inhabitants, doesn't support a radiotherapy unit, but this pattern of events is repeated every day around the world in equally wealthy countries with large rural areas and difficult access to the nearest major city. Furthermore, in the poorest countries in the world, the women with early breast cancer can't even be offered BCS because of the inadequacy in the provision of radiotherapy centres. Assuming there never will be a golden age when all women in the world, suffering with breast cancer have easy access to post operative radiotherapy, we need some original thinking "outside the box" to offer a solution. If the woman can't get to the radiotherapy unit then the radiotherapy unit must come to the woman. I now wish to describe the rationale, the technique and the results of trials that may indeed answer the problem with a simple mobile radiotherapy unit. This unit (INTRABEAM) can provide a one shot intra-operative treatment (IORT) targeting the area around the primary tumour, that has been accepted as being equivalent to 5 to 7 weeks of conventional external beam treatment in selected cases. The rationale for targeting the area around the primary tumour comes from clinical correlation of whole organ analysis of mastectomy specimens. It has been well demonstrated that the female breast frequently harbours more than one tumour and these are found if one looks hard enough. They have been demonstrated in autopsy studies- up to 20% of women with a median age of 39 [16] as well as in mastectomy specimens [17]. However, their widespread 3-dimensional distribution does not correspond to the location of recurrences after breast conserving surgery [18, 19], which occurs most commonly (about 90%) in the area around the scar of primary excision (index quadrant). Hence it follows that radiotherapy after surgical excision should be targeted to the area around the primary tumour- the tumour bed. Conventional external beam radiotherapy is very successful and reduces the rate of local recurrence by 2/3rds- but that means it fails in 1/3 of cases. This could be because of intrinsic resistance of any residual cancer cells, or due to the radiotherapy dose "geographically" missing the target tissues and "temporally" missing the window of optimal opportunity. It is interesting that the proportional reduction of the risk does not change with increasing size of excision. Hence just excising the cancer with a larger margin will not eliminate the risk. As IORT is delivered immediately after surgery it may avoid both the geographical and temporal missing of the target.

In 1998 my department at UCL pioneered the approach of *targ*eted *i*ntraoperative radio*t*herapy (TARGIT) [20, 21]. With our technique, using the Intrabeam™ system, a single fraction of 20Gy is delivered to the surface of the tumour bed using a spherical applicator, from within the breast. The surgeon "wraps" (or conforms) the pliable tumour bed around the applicator, ensuring close apposition of the target tissue to the radiotherapy source. The technique needs to be meticulous but is relatively straightforward and so far over 4,000 patients have been treated worldwide. Although the approach of concentrating on the tumour bed is not new, modern technology has allowed it to be used with relative ease in a routine operating theatre and with a potential for significant economic saving.

After successful completion of a pilot study [21], we launched the Targit A trial in March 2000. In this trial, we selected women who were older than 45 years and those who did not face a high risk of developing recurrent or multiple cancers in the breast. In fact, these women form the majority of breast cancer patients. The randomly allocated treatment that followed wide excision of the cancer (lumpectomy) was either targeted IORT or the usual 3 to 6 week course of external beam radiotherapy. The aim of the trial was modest- to investigate if the two treatments were equivalent- but if proven, the prize was great- women could then avoid the 30-40 visits to the radiotherapy centre and still conserve their breast. The results of the TARGIT A trial in terms of safety, efficacy and patient satisfaction have now published [22] Furthermore evidence in support of its adoption for carefully selected cases emerges from a number of consensus statements that include one from the American Society of Breast Cancer Surgeons and one from the biennial European St Gallen conference. [23, 24]

This most recent and in many ways the most exciting example of the transfer of appropriate technology, has been the establishment of the first unit in Thailand for delivering intra-operative radiotherapy (IORT) after breast conserving surgery, here at the Queen Sikirit breast cancer centre in Bangkok. We can now witness the true meaning of globalization at its best: The invention of a miniature electron generator/accelerator in Boston MA, incorporated into a mobile Xray treatment unit by Carl Zeiss in Germany, pioneered for the single dose treatment of breast cancer by a team based at University College London, and tested in a multinational clinical trial in 11 countries means we can now offer Thai women who live too far from a radiotherapy centre, to enjoy the benefits of breast conserving surgery, with a stay of one day rather than six weeks in the big city. Our future vision is to provide one of these mobile units on a railway train to travel up and down the country acting as a mobile education and treatment centre. The fulfilment of this vision now depends on political will rather than technology transfer.

That aside we can take comfort from the fact that Globalization of scientific endeavour can improve both length of life and quality of life for at least one common cancer type anywhere in the world but no doubt others will follow the path beaten by breast cancer pioneers. All that the masters of our universe have to do to achieve this ambition is to remember the biblical injunction:

Thou shalt love thy neighbour as thy self.

References

[1] Moynihan R. Surrogates under scrutiny. *BMJ* 2011, 343:399-401.

[2] Priestman TJ, Baum M. Evaluation of quality of life in patients receiving treatment for advanced breast cancer. *Lancet* 1976;i:899-901

[3] Montazeri A. Health-related quality of life in breast cancer patients: a bibliographic review of the literature from 1974 to 2007. *J Exp Clin Cancer Res.* 2008 Aug 29;27:32.

[4] Dhillon PK, Yeole BB, Dikshit R, Kurkure AP, Bray F. Trends in breast, ovarian and cervical cancer incidence in Mumbai, India over a 30-year period, 1976-2005: an age-period-cohort analysis. *Br J Cancer.* 2011.301: 1038.

[5] Autier P, Boniol M, Gavin A, Vatten LJ, Breast cancer mortality in neighbouring European countries with different levels of screening but similar access to treatment: trend analysis of WHO mortality database. *BMJ*, 2011, 343:300.

[6] Jørgensen KJ, Gøtzsche PC. Overdiagnosis in publicly organised mammography screening programmes: systematic review of incidence trends. *BMJ* 2009;338-341.
[7] Welch GH, Black WC. Over-diagnosis in cancer. *J Natl Cancer Inst.* 2010;102:605-13.
[8] Welch, HG, Screening mammography - A long run for a short slide? *N Engl J Med.* 2010;363:13.
[9] McPherson K. Should we screen for breast cancer? *BMJ* 2010;341:233-5.
[10] US Preventive Services Task Force. Screening for breast cancer: recommendation statement. *Ann Int Med* 2009;151:716-26.
[11] Gøtzsche PC, Nielsen M. Screening for breast cancer with mammography. *Cochrane Database Syst Rev* 2009;4:CD001877.
[12] Baum M. Biological considerations in the management of early carcinoma of the breast and their role in the selection of therapy. *Ann Roy Col Surg Engl* 1980;62:35-38.
[13] Fisher B, Anderson S, Bryant J, et al. Twenty-year follow-up of a randomized trial comparing total mastectomy, lumpectomy, and lumpectomy plus irradiation for the treatment of invasive breast cancer. *N Engl J Med* 2002;347:1233-41.
[14] Early Breast Cancer Trialists' Collaborative Group (EBCTCG). Effects of chemotherapy and hormonal therapy for early breast cancer on recurrence and 15 year survival: an overview of the randomised trials. *Lancet* 2005; 365: 1687-1717.
[15] Jones A, Ellis P. Potential withdrawal of bevacizumab for the treatment of breast cancer ,BMJ 2011;343:1136.
[16] Nielsen M, Thomsen JL, Primdahl S, Dyreborg U, Andersen JA: Breast cancer and atypia among young and middle-aged women: a study of 110 medicolegal autopsies. *Br J Cancer* 56:814-819, 1987.
[17] Holland R, Veling SH, Mravunac M, Hendriks JH: Histologic multifocality of Tis, T1-2 breast carcinomas. Implications for clinical trials of breast-conserving surgery. *Cancer* 56:979-990, 1985.
[18] Vaidya JS, Vyas JJ, Mittra I, Chinoy RF: Multicentricity and its influence on conservative breast cancer treatment strategy. *Hongkong International Cancer Congress: Abstract* 44.4, 1995.
[19] Baum M, Vaidya JS, Mittra I: Multicentricity and recurrence of breast cancer [letter; comment]. *Lancet* 349:208, 1997.

[20] Vaidya JS: A novel approach for local treatment of early breast cancer. PhD Thesis, University of London: http://www.dundee.ac.uk/~jsvaidya/papers/thesis.htm, 2002.

[21] Vaidya JS, Baum M, Tobias JS, D'Souza DP, Naidu SV, Morgan S, Metaxas M, Harte KJ, Sliski AP, Thomson E: Targeted intra-operative radiotherapy (Targit): an innovative method of treatment for early breast cancer. *Ann Oncol* 12:1075-1080, 2001.

[22] Vaidya JS, Baum M, Tobias JS, Morgan S, D'Souza D: The novel technique of delivering targeted intraoperative radiotherapy (Targit) for early breast cancer. *Eur J Surg Oncol* 28:447-454, 2000.

[23] Vaidya JS, Joseph DJ, et al.: Targeted intraoperative radiotherapy versus whole breast radiotherapy for breast cancer (TARGIT-A trial): an international, prospective, randomised, non-inferiority phase 3 trial. *Lancet* 2010; 376; 91-102.

[24] The American Society of Breast Surgeons: Consensus Statement for Accelerated Partial Breast Irradiation. Revised 2008. http://www.breastsurgeons.org/statements /index.php

[25] Goldhirsch A, Wood WC, et al.: Strategies for subtypes – dealing with the diversity of breast cancer: highlights of the St Gallen International Expert Consensus on the Primary Therapy of Early Breast Cancer 2011. Annals of Oncology Advance Access; 2011.

Chapter 5

Ethical Issues in Screening for Cancer

Modern medicine is a minefield of ethical dilemmas ranging from stem cell research, in vitro fertilization, termination of pregnancy, consent for treatment, consent for clinical trials and end of life decisions concerning withholding treatment or even euthanasia. When analyzing these problems the scholarly medical ethicist tends to fall back on the teachings of Immanuel Kant and his concepts of the categorical imperatives of human relationships in a democratic society.

> "Finally, there is an imperative which commands a certain conduct immediately, without having as its condition any other purpose to be attained by it. This imperative is Categorical. This imperative may be called that of Morality"
>
> Grundlegung zur Metaphysik der Sitten ,section II

These teachings were translated into the ethical standards of modern medicine by the classic work of Beauchamp and Childress, *Principles of Biomedical Ethics, OUP 1989,* known as the four principles. These can be listed as follows:

- Beneficence (the obligation to provide benefits and balance benefits against risks).
- Non-maleficence (the obligation to avoid the causation of harm)

- Respect for autonomy (the obligation to respect the decision making capacities of autonomous persons)
- Justice (the obligation of fairness in the distribution of benefits and risks).

To which I would like to add a fifth:

- Distributive justice (the obligation to ensure that scarce resources are distributed fairly amongst the health services for the greatest health improvement for the greatest number)

This "Utilitarian" principle is an extension of the teachings of Jeremy Bentham, the founder of University College London (1748-1832) who argued for the greatest good for the greatest number. *"Everybody to count for one, nobody for more than one."* However, this principle can be interpreted in two ways. Firstly public health interventions where something is done to the whole community for the benefit of the "public health", and secondly in the rationing of health care so that the greatest cost/utility is achieved for the greatest number in the allocation of a finite health expenditure.

Unfortunately it is never easy to achieve moral equilibrium. The greatest ethical dilemmas in medicine follow on from a clash of these high sounding ethical imperatives.

It is my contention that the subject of screening for cancer has been allowed to drift into accepted public health practice without the appropriate vigorous ethical debate we have witnessed for the subjects I've listed above.

In discussing the ethical issues of screening for cancer we must accept a tension that exists between "Utilitarian" principles of public health and that of the "Autonomy" of the individual imposed upon. Utilitarianism involves social engineering for the "greatest good of the greatest number", whereas autonomy assumes that the individual has an informed choice when health interventions for "their own good" are considered. Social engineering and coercion might be acceptable for hygiene and substance abuse, but when the balance of benefit versus harm is a close call then surely the right to self -determination trumps the principle of utilitarianism. Nowhere is this truer than in the area of mammographic screening for breast cancer. We screen for breast cancer to reduce cause-specific mortality without an increase in all cause mortality and at an acceptable cost in terms of medical morbidity, i.e. in the name of beneficence. At the same time we should also consider whether the costs of such programs might be spent in better ways to improve the health care in the community or at least achieve the same objectives, i.e. in the name of distributive justice. Even if we accept uncritically the results of the randomized controlled trials as evidence for a reduction in cancer specific mortality, the benefit in absolute risk reduction is so small (widely accepted as 1:10,000 woman years of screening over the age of 50 and about 1:15,000 woman years of screening for the younger age groups) then the individual woman should have the right to make a personal trade off against the undoubted harms of false alarms, over-diagnosis and radical treatments for diseases that, if left to nature would never announce themselves in a natural lifetime. I therefore propose that the uncritical promotion of screening as illustrated by the high profile government campaigns to induce women to accept mammographic screening, is unethical by modern standards and reflects a paternalistic attitude that would be unacceptable for treatment of the established disease or for entry into clinical trials. In other words we are witnessing a double standard at play with screening for cancer enjoying a "privileged" position.

Finally in the name of distributive justice I also believe that in UK at least we should have an open debate about the expenditure of the £100,000,000 a year on the NHSBSP which some might think might be better spent on Cinderella specialties, such as care of the elderly or at least in the reduction of the waiting list for postoperative radiotherapy for breast cancer which might save as many lives as screening.

I have a sneaking suspicion here that there is a political agenda here, not only for the UK but also for the rest of Europe. Screening demonstrates that governments are "doing something about breast cancer", whereas other uses of the same money do not win votes.

Chapter 6

The Use and Abuse of Human Tissue: An Analysis of the Ethical Issues Raised by the Proposed Human Tissue Act

Medico Legal Journal.2004;72 (Pt 2):67-9.

Historical Introduction

There has been a shift in our attitudes to the nature of "Human tissue" over the history of mankind. This can roughly be divided into four eras: pre-biblical paganism, the biblical period up to the 18thC, the "Age of enlightenment" up to the late 20thC and the modern era that demonstrates a confusing amalgam of cultural relativism, religious fundamentalism and neo-paganism (new-ageism).

A few examples may illuminate this point. In ancient Egyptian burial ritual it was apparent that, at least for the wealthy, the after-life continued in a bodily form similar to that on earth. For this reason the deceased's body had to be preserved from decay and sent on its journey with all his or her worldly goods.

In contrast the Judeo/Christian belief system taught that the afterlife was a spiritual domain or as Maimonides, the great 12thC doctor and philosopher put it: "There are neither bodies nor bodily forms in the world to come but only the disembodied souls of the righteous who have become like the ministering Angels". Yet in spite of this, the teaching of all the great monotheistic religions are that "man was created in God's image", therefore the body and even body parts have to be treated with respect and wherever possible buried intact.

The great thinkers of the age of enlightenment like Montaigne, Voltaire and Bentham took a much more sceptical and pragmatic approach to the body and its parts. For example Jeremy Bentham, founder of the philosophical school of "Utilitarianism" and founder of University College London, believed that "The happiness of the greatest number is the measure of right or wrong". With this in mind he advocated that the empty husk of a dead body was of greater value as an aid in teaching anatomy than buried six feet under. He set an example and his post-dissected, reconstructed, embalmed and fashionably dressed body is still on view at the entrance to UCL on Gower Street.

A Modern "Scandal"

The current controversy and confusion on the proper disposal of human tissue results from this inheritance from the past coupled with a volatile stew of belief systems ranging from post-modern relativism to religious fundamentalism with a healthy dose of neo-paganism as tragically witnessed in the procession of mini-coffins containing children's body parts after the Bristol and Alder-Hey scandals.

It is my concern that the justifiable response to reassure the public after these unforgivable excesses, in the drafting of the human tissue act, is in danger of over reaction and by the "law of unintended consequences" could lead to preventable tragedies in the future.

Why do doctors wish to retain body parts or human tissue?

To read some of the hysterical reactions in the tabloid press you would think that most doctors are ghouls! It would also appear that there is a lot of ignorance why the medical profession legitimately needs access to body parts and human tissue.

A few of the legitimate reasons can be listed as follows:

- To teach Anatomy for undergraduates and surgeons.
- To teach Pathology.
- For the diagnosis of cause of death at autopsy.

- For medical audit.
- For research.

At the same time one can sympathize with the lay public and bereaved relatives in confusing these activities with freak shows. There is a legitimate hierarchy in the use and abuse of body parts which can be described as the "yuck" index which can be ranked as follows:

- Deformed fetuses in bottles.
- Normal organs in bottles.
- Diseased organs in bottles.
- Surgical specimens in bottles.
- Tumors in bottles.
- Wax blocks of diseased tissue from archive.
- Pathology slides from archive.
- Cell cultures of human origin.
- DNA
- Serum
- Urine
- Sputum

It therefore takes cool heads and mature judgment where to draw the line even if we assume that the laws of data protection are respected in each case.

A Question of Ownership

The subject becomes even more complicated when you consider the concept of ownership. First of all we must respect the metaphysical/spiritual belief that our bodies are the property of our creator in whose image we are cast. In which case no one "owns" the body of the deceased. We then have to consider the Kantian philosophy that the right to self- determination or autonomy trumps all other ethical premises. If that is the case then ***we*** "own" our bodies and can use them as we wish: yet there is a moral inconsistency here, in that it is considered unethical to sell ones blood or kidneys. We even have a legal debate on the issue as to whether it is theft to dig up a body that can be deemed abandoned after death. This analysis reflects that what we are witnessing is a conflict of different models of moral philosophy: Deism

/Religiosity, Utilitarianism and Kantian autonomy. Without a clear understanding of this we are doomed to make a serious mistake with the hasty implementation of the human tissue act.

The Law of Unintended Consequences

Before it is too late we must ask ourselves some serious questions.

In the name of preventing a further Bristol or Alder-Hey scandal are we prepared to risk any of the following?

- Inadequately trained doctors who have no spatial understanding of human anatomy or who cannot recognize the features of morbid anatomy.
- Loss of medical audit whereby the ante-mortem diagnoses are checked against the post-mortem findings. Here we have another paradox in that the very practices we need to strengthen to prevent another "Shipman tragedy" * would be impeded by too great a respect for the body of the deceased.
- Do we want to make some varieties of cancer research impossible? Although this is a rhetorical question we can in fact illustrate this with a real and active problem.

I was principle investigator of the ATAC trial. This study recruited over 9,000 patients with early breast cancer, comparing the adjuvant use of tamoxifen and the aromatase inhibitor, arimidex. This study demonstrated an advantage of arimidex over tamoxifen in both efficacy and tolerability. Since this study started, new data emerged that suggested that patients whose tumors over-expressed the Her2-neu antigen might be the ones who enjoyed this advantage and offered us a real choice for the individualization of therapy. Unfortunately because of the current EU guidelines we have to re-consent all our volunteers to study this biomarker on their archival material. This in itself is costly and time consuming forgetting the fact that the most important cases are those women who have already had a recurrence many of whom have died. Yet when approached individually these women think it is absurd and express no residual interest in the sanctity of their stored malignant tissue.

One can only guess at the magnitude of the problem the two year delay has caused to thousands of women world wide who may have been under or over treated as a result of this bureaucratic delay.

Conclusion

The question we must therefore answer is how best to protect the public from the abuses of the past; accommodate all the ethical and religious beliefs that co-exist in a vibrant multicultural society, whilst maintaining medical standards and encouraging legitimate research. We could make a good start by legally defining all biopsy and surgical specimens as donations [1]. Next, anonymizing all human material in research databases whilst accepting a legal requirement for autopsy as the default position, all of which would protect scientific progress and audit. Finally the deceased's family request for burial or cremation without a post mortem must then be treated with respect and sensitivity, providing they can demonstrate legitimate ethical or religious grounds and in the absence of suspicious circumstances.

* Dr. Harold Shipman, an English General Practitioner and mass murderer

Reference

[1] Biopsy specimens should be legally defined as donations, Wright PK, *BMJ* 2004, 328;642.

Chapter 7

"Playing God - Jewish Perspectives on Cloning and Genetic Engineering"

Rabbi Breitowitz
Associate Professor of Law at the University of Maryland and the Rabbi of the Woodside Synagogue in Silver Spring, Maryland
(Review for Jewish Renaissance)

I approached this lecture with some trepidation preparing to disagree violently with any Rabbi who was prepared to pass judgment on these complex scientific and ethical issues. On seeing the speaker for the first time my adrenalin levels started to rise as the Rabbi appeared to be a clone of all the other black hated and bearded Rabbis who have angered me in the past. Yet within five minutes I was totally won over. I was hanging on his every word and this Jew who prides himself on being of the secular wing of his faith concluded that being orthodox Jewish, wasn't all bad! For a start he provided us with a beautiful eulogy on the late Chief Rabbi, Lord Jacobovits. I knew the late Chief Rabbi extremely well and loved him dearly. I was even proud to be a member of his kitchen cabinet, which met regularly in the Jakobovits' household's kitchen to discuss medical ethics. Rabbi Breitowitz described the late Chief Rabbi as choosing the path of truth rather than the path of peace. In other word was far from politically correct. With this I agreed wholeheartedly and this was probably the reason I held the late great Chief Rabbi in such high esteem even though I often disagreed with him.

For a start Rabbi Breitowitz promised that he would not offer a halachic solution to the problem. A Rabbi without a solution – my kind of Rabbi!

He then proceeded to contrast the Jewish approach to the Christian Science approach in response to medical progress. Whereas the Christian Scientists believe that as God delivers disease so it should be left to God to deliver its cure and if the patient dies then surely that is God's will; Judaism totally rejects this passivity and believes that there is a divine licence to practice the medical arts. The philosophical underpinning for this belief is that wisdom and understanding are gifts of God to be used as part of God's plan. Rabbi Breitowitz quoted Rabbi Akivah who claimed that God left creation incomplete and it was the gift of God for us to use our wisdom and understanding to improve on creation. In other words Man *is supposed* to play God! Well that was a knockout blow early on in his discourse, by which time I was sitting on the edge of my seat wondering what on earth could come next.

He then went on to discuss a 12th Century debate between Rambam & Rashi concerning whether or not the lay public should have access to a book on the practice of medicine. Rashi applied the "American Medical Association" interpretation on this, in other words protecting the closed shop. But the Rambam, as always humane in his interpretation, agreed that the lay public should be denied access to medical literature in order to prevent self-medication in the absence of adequate evidence. In other words Maimonides (Rabbi Moishe ben Maimom) had anticipated the evidence based medicine movement by about 800 years or putting it another way, the rabbinical age of enlightenment anticipated the European movement by about 500 years.

Rabbi Breitowitz then went on to define two types of cloning: reproductive, to produce another human being; or therapeutic, to provide a source of stem cells. In discussing this he demonstrated a masterful understanding of cell and molecular biology, pointing out that in theory sperm would not be necessary for reproduction in the future because women would be able to clone themselves. I assumed that the wise Rabbi would immediately reject the notion of cloning a human being but this was not to be the case. He offered us a thought experiment. Say there was a wise and virtuous man who was the last in the line of a great family, all of whom had died in the Holocaust, and say he had been castrated by the Nazis, then he and his wife might have a legitimate wish to continue the family line using the cytoplasm from one of her eggs, the nuclear material from one of his somatic cells and re-implanting the embryo into his wife's womb. Having convinced us that we should not automatically reject the notion of cloning for reproduction, he then described some of the generic concerns on the ethics of this future technology before getting down to specific halachic issues.

- Human cloning will be an expensive and scarce resource. In the USA, market forces will then determine who should be cloned. Whereas in the UK the pressures will be rationalised, no doubt to produce socially desirable individuals, which is another word for eugenics.
- What about quality control? If human beings are seen as a commodity what happens to the failures that have serious genetic defects?
- What about the psychological burden of being a clone? – The poor clone would have lost some of his individuality and autonomy, after all biology is not destiny
- The creation of a clone separates love from the creation of life
- If cloning oneself becomes a reality then our awareness of the finite limit of life will be perturbed with unpredictable social consequences.

Coming now to the Halachic issues:

- First of all there are the lineage problems – is the clone a real human being or a golem. Does the clone therefore inherit?
- Is my clone my son or my brother? If he is my brother and should I die then according to Halachic tradition he should be offered first refusal on my widow who would be his mother!
- How many clones does it take to make a *mynyan*? (A quorum of 10 Jewish men over the age of 13 required for a Jewish service.)
- If the man takes the nucleus from a somatic cell and implants it into the ovary of a non-Jewish woman is the child Jewish or not? The issue becomes even more complex when a woman decides to clone herself using one of her somatic nuclei implanted into the cytoplasm of another woman's egg and the embryo implanted into another woman's uterus.

Admittedly some of these scenarios were extremely unlikely and extremely amusing but at the same time of such far-reaching importance they have to be taken seriously. Coming on to therapeutic cloning, the issues were a little bit simpler. The Halachic tradition is extremely lenient about abortion prior to forty days of gestation. In other words external embryonic development in vitro up to this point is not considered to be an interference with latent life. Furthermore therapeutic cloning of an individual's embryo for their own stem cells gets round most, if not all of the theoretical halachic problems. Best of all though was to encourage work on the mechanisms by which it would be possible to switch on the appropriate DNA sequences in a terminally differentiated somatic cell that would allow it to develop into specific organs in vitro, bypassing the need for an embryo stage or as Rabbi Breitowitz put it; "from my hand to my heart"

As I pointed out in the discussion this was not all that far fetched. There is a natural experiment by which apparently terminally differentiated cells revert to a pluri-potential phenotype. This is when we observe cancer cells undergoing "metaplasia." Examples include bladder epithelial cells transforming themselves into skin-like squamous epithelium or breast cancer cells transforming themselves into sweat glands.

I came into the room secure in my belief that **man** had created God, prepared to challenge Rabbi Breitowitz in his belief that **God** had created man. I left the room an hour later realising that both sets of belief were compatible. Never have I experienced a lecture that has so transformed me and convinced me that to be a Jew does not demand the abdication of the mind.

Medical Humanities

Chapter 8

The Re-Emerging Role of the Humanities in the Education of Medical Undergraduates

(Address to the Royal College of Physicians 2001, published in Clinical Medicine, 2002, 2; 246 -249)

Introduction

Amongst the many German doctors indicted at Nuremberg for crimes against humanity in 1946, where tenured Professors, clinical Directors, personal physicians, the Head of the German Red Cross and bio-medical researchers employed by the pharmaceutical industry. [1] Some of the leading physicians amongst Germany's medical establishment even committed suicide before their interrogation or indictment. Many of these were considered men of refined culture. The music of Wagner and Beethoven was often broadcast over the loudspeakers in the concentration camps. It can thus be seen that culture alone does not make for a humane physician and the function of teaching arts and humanities to medical under-graduates is not so that they will enjoy a night at the opera when they qualify, but to ensure that they make better and more humane physicians who are instinctively appalled by human suffering and do everything within their power, even to the point of significant self-sacrifice, to save a life or to succour someone in mortal pain.

It is the purpose of this paper to provide some justification for the teaching of arts and humanities to medical students. I have arrived at these conclusions after some twenty-five years as a medical educator, twenty years spent at professorial level. During this time I have had academic responsibilities at three of our great National medical Schools. I have had a central role in the curriculum development at the Welsh National School of Medicine, King's College School of Medicine & Dentistry and the Royal Free & University College London Medical Schools. In addition, for a number of years I was Chairman of the con-joint examination Board in Surgery for the University of London.

During this time I have witnessed the ever-expanding knowledge base that we are trying to impose on our students, with an ever-worsening ratio of staff to student numbers. The developments of cell and molecular biology, which impact on all human disease processes, is taking an increasing share of our curriculum time with the ever-present danger that molecular reductionism may somehow leave the whole patient behind. Yet as a clinician and a scientist I want to resist falling into the popular trap of post-modern relativism in rejecting the scientific method in favour of some vague metaphysical notion of "holistic" medicine.

At the same time I share a view with many of my senior academic colleagues that there is a real danger of losing the humanity in the practice of medicine by ignoring many of the subjects that are conventionally taught within the Faculties of Arts and Humanities. I believe with great fervour that the teaching of arts and humanities, in addition to ensuring that our young doctors practice in an ethical and humane way, will paradoxically enhance their understanding of science and improve their communication skills, thus transforming them into better diagnosticians, whilst improving the satisfaction of their patient clients.

HOW ARTS AND HUMANITIES CAN CONTRIBUTE TO THE SCIENCE & PRACTICE OF MEDICINE

Science and the Arts are the twin pillars upon which our Western cultural heritage is supported; yet little progress has been made since CP Snow's seminal essays of the 1960's demonstrated the separation of these two cultures. [3] The polarization of these two bodies of knowledge is perpetuated by our education system to the impoverishment of all. Even the best educated amongst our political and academic leaders have lost close on 50% of their cultural inheritance and the Renaissance man has all but disappeared from modern Society.

Revolutionary thinking about an undergraduate medical curriculum may see the profession of medicine as the natural bonding medium between these two cultures. This would not only be of value for the individual doctor but inevitably for the patient he treats and ultimately for Society as a whole.

Yet before we get carried away in our derogation of the scientist let us remember that the members of the arts faculties are equally illiterate in the understanding of science. It is therefore fair to quote the following passage from an essay by Melvyn Bragg: "It is impossible to be educated today in an advanced Society and confess to a lack of knowledge or interest in science .... It is obvious to me that scientists know far more about the arts than arts people know about the sciences" [4]

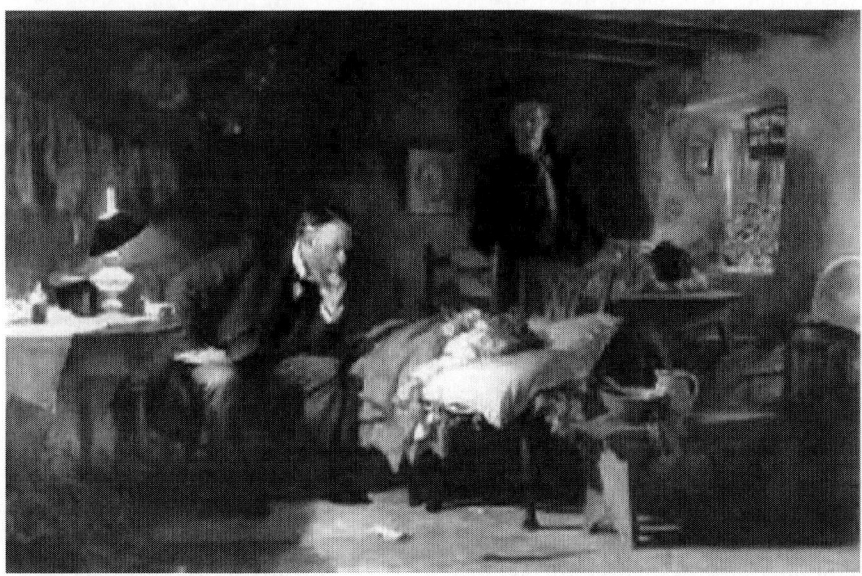

The Doctor, by Sir Luke Fildes, 1901.

The spectacular advances over the last two decades in the development of recombinant technology, the decoding of the human genome, and the technology of molecular research, have contributed to the advancement of science; yet have deconstructed the human subject to a molecular level. Inevitably, better understanding of human disease and better treatments will emerge from this process and in itself I have no argument against this degree of reductionism. Unfortunately, we have so far been unable to reconstitute the complex organism of the human being up through the various hierarchical levels to that of a successful and healthy personality existing comfortably within his own Society. I think it is an exaggeration to argue that this reductionism resulting from molecular biology has led to the brutalisation of medicine, but certainly it has done nothing to contribute to the humanisation of our subject.

Paradoxically, when treatments were least effective the humanitarian instinct of the doctor was virtually all that was on offer. You have only got to read the romance of "Dr Finlay's casebook" or to look at the painting "The doctor" by Sir Luke Fildes in The Tate Britain, to appreciate this fact. Yet as treatments become more effective and the pace of change increases in the new millennium, doctors are in danger of losing their humanitarian instincts to become mere technocrats, often expressing arrogance in their wish to medicalize aspects of human behaviour that are strictly none of the doctors' business.

Why Arts Courses for Medical Students?

This was the question posed by Sir Kenneth Calman (Chief Medical Officer) and Professor Robin Downie of the Department of Philosophy of the University of Glasgow, in their editorial in the Lancet on June 1st 1996 [5].

I would like to quote one paragraph from this commentary, which I believe sets the scene. "Unlike Science which is concerned with the general, the repeatable elements in nature, medicine albeit using science, is concerned with the uniqueness of individual patients. In its concern for the particular and the unique, medicine resembles the Arts. In its concentration on the repeatable patterns and laws of nature, science must of necessity be impersonal". Professor Robin Downie has done more than pay lip service in his beliefs, but has pioneered a special study module for the humanising of medicine at the University of Glasgow.

I believe that the Arts/Science dichotomy in the practice of Medicine is entirely fallacious as both are integral to the skilled practice of modern medicine. I say this not out of political correctness (I am most certainly not "feely-touchy") but out of a hard-nosed pragmatic view based on 25 years experience as a clinical scientist.

I would briefly like to discuss the practical applications of philosophy, theology, literature\theatre, fine art and music for the enhancement of medical education.

Philosophy of Science

Although it is often tempting to search amongst the thinkers of the ancient orient for enlightenment and wisdom, we should also be proud of our Western heritage for scientific philosophy. Science as a philosophy was founded once in the history of mankind in the golden age of Pericles in ancient Greece, and the development of science as a philosophy can be traced from Aristotle via the age of enlightenment in Western Europe, to the late 20th Century. To this day we often describe our teaching methods as Socratic when we encourage students to think for themselves rather than handing down received wisdom. Our Western tradition of philosophy has emphasised that scepticism is a healthy attribute. For example, Maimonides (12th C. Alexandria) had the dictum "teach your tongue to say I do not know and thou shalt progress". The essays of Michel de Montaigne (16th C, France) taught us to develop an antithesis when anyone wished to impose the received wisdom on contemporary thinking. He even went so far in one essay as to ask the distasteful question "what is fundamentally wrong with cannibalism?" A similar collection of essays were published by our own Sir Thomas Browne of 17th C Norwich, a famous physician of his time, who dared to question the holy bible by pointing out that from his research, men and women had the same number of ribs and therefore it was highly unlikely that the first man lost his twelfth rib on the left hand side in order to produce the first woman! However, the greatest richness in the history of science and philosophy emerges from the British School of thought, which illustrated the poverty of Artistotelian inductivism. This can be attributed largely to the writings of Hume, the Scottish 18th C philosopher, and developed further in the 20th Century by Sir Bertrand Russell and Sir Karl Popper.

Evidence Based Medicine

These days we talk about evidence-based medicine as if we truly understand what this means, yet it is accepted that the gold standard for evidence-based medicine are the results from reproducible randomised controlled trials. How many proponents of the randomised controlled trial appreciate that Popper's "Logic of Scientific Discovery" codified the philosophical underpinning for this approach? (6). Yet it must not be forgotten that some of the most important developments in the history of medicine, such as the discovery of penicillin or insulin, were not dependent on the conventional modern standards required for evidence based medicine. Undergraduates and postgraduates alike need to appreciate the poverty of inductivism, the fertility of deductivism, whilst seeing the history of medicine as a series of paradigm shifts as described by the late Thomas Kuhn [7]

Perhaps the most dramatic paradigm shift in the history of medicine (which ultimately led to the death of Galenic doctrine) was the demonstration of the circulation of the blood by William Harvey who predicted that there had to be invisible channels linking the arterial and venous systems, approximately one hundred years before Antoni van Leeuwenhoek invented the microscope, which in due course was able to demonstrate these structures. That was a spectacular corroboration of Harvey's predictions that incidentally demonstrates that falsificationism alone is not the only way to acquire wisdom. Sadly we witness today the growth in the interest of alternative medicine, which in many cases is a return to the teachings of Galen. An intelligent young medical student armed with knowledge of the history and philosophy of science, should be able to make the demarcation between scientific (rational) medicine versus unscientific irrational or alternative medicine. At the same time it would be a foolish and inhumane young student who threw out the baby with the bath water.

Holistic Medicine

We have many lessons to learn from the growing enthusiasm for alternative medicine amongst the lay public. Jan Smuts coined the word "holism" in 1926. He used the word to describe the tendency in nature to create wholes from ordered groupings of units. In other words, the whole is greater than the sum of parts. The holistic model of the human being is a valuable concept but the naïve ideas expressed as the three-legged stool (mind, body and spirit) are insufficient to take account of the modern understanding of biology and physiology. It is indeed possible to reconstruct the whole person upwards through a hierarchical system exactly as described in Robert

Pirsig's cult book "Zen and the Art of the Motorcycle Maintenance" [8], or taking this to a more sophisticated level using the notion of the holon as described by Arthur Koestler in the "Ghost in the Machine" [9]. Using this model we can reconstruct the human being from autonomous sub-cellular components such as mitochondria, to the single cell, to cells acting in concert within an organ, for organs co-operating together orchestrated via circulating hormones and lymphocytes to the psyche situated somewhere in the brain, acting on the soma through cortico/hypothalamic pathways, to the highest level of activity of the human subject in sickness and health.

Students need to understand the value of qualitative research, "they need to get down from their veranda and mix with the natives". Students need to learn the importance of measuring social adjustment and quality of life, and that these outcome measures maybe as important as of length of life. We need to acknowledge the contributions of alternative medicine in reminding us of the importance of studying these subjective outcomes, yet at the same time we must not court popularity with unquestioning acceptance of many of these bizarre health belief systems which are patently absurd. (10) Any intervention dreamed up by human kind has the capacity for benefit and harm. The scientific method is sufficiently robust to study subjective outcomes and quality of life in trials of any intervention whether it originates from the main stream or the fringe.

Philosophy and Theology in Relation to the Understanding and Teaching of Medical Ethics

Medical ethics are not absolute codes of conduct that leapt fully formed and immutable from the heads of ancient sages in distant times. Medical ethics in fact demonstrate an uncomfortable plasticity with subtle variations emerging between different ages in history and between different ethnic and cultural groups. Medical ethics may be driven by the law of the land or by medical technology, but more often than not medical technology runs in advance of our capacity for ethical control. But the law is a blunt instrument that may belatedly react to some of the worst medical abuses or as a late reaction to public outcry. All ethical codes of conduct for the practice of medicine have their bedrock in philosophy and theology. For example, the Hippocratic oath, which is seldom recited today, probably emerged as a result of the teachings of respect for human rights and dignity at the time of democracy in Athens 400 years before the Common Era. Much of the teaching of Plato and Socrates can be seen reflected in the teachings of Hippocrates. In contrast, contemporary medical ethics is heavily dependent on the teachings of Immanuel Kant of the 19th Century AD which have been translated into the four "categorical imperatives" of Beauchamp and Childress [11] – autonomy, beneficence, non-maleficence and justice. Contemporary medical problems illustrate the tensions that arise when there is often a clash of these categorical imperatives, particularly between distributive justice on one hand and the right to autonomy or self-determination on the other. Furthermore, some of these "categorical imperatives" clash with ethnic or religious minorities. For example, an absolute belief in the right to self-determination would encourage suicide and assisted euthanasia that would be an anathema to orthodox Jewish teaching. The Jewish faith believes that life is of infinite value and you cannot split infinity. Therefore every moment of life is of infinite value, and therefore the individual or the doctor working on the individual's instruction must not do anything to shorten life. In a similar way, witness the current furore regarding the debate between the anti-abortionist (who describe themselves as pro-lifers) and those demanding the freedom of the individual to control their families by the use of abortion where necessary (pro-choice). According to Roman Catholic doctrine, life begins at conception and the individual does not have sufficient autonomy to end the life of the unborn child. Thus, even within our narrow Western world of Judeo-Christian belief system, there are many tensions. Yet when we recognise that our Society exhibits an enormous range of cultural and religious diversity, the problems are magnified. For example, how do we accommodate the Shariah law of Islam and the Hindu systems of caste and belief in reincarnation? Once again we are in danger of losing respect for minorities within our pluralistic Society, whilst on the other hand drifting guiltily into a post-modern relativism of "anything goes". Our young doctors must learn to respect and celebrate the ethnic and cultural diversity of the Society in which they work, and therefore need to study the fundamentals of theological belief shared by large numbers of their prospective patients.

Of course, theology plays a much more important role in Society than merely underpinning our code of medical ethics. Theology is the basis of faith and faith provides spiritual solace for our patients at the time of suffering and when confronting the inevitability of death. The practice of religion can contribute to the healing of the spirit, but a clear demarcation has to be made from spiritual healing and healing of the body, although we must leave room to speculate on the links that might exist between a spirit at peace with itself and a body best equipped to heal itself. [12] Nevertheless, from my own experience in oncology, I must warn my students of the quackery that finds fertile soil in filling the gaps vacated by faith in an essentially secular Society. The "new age" belief systems have led to a return to animism, idolatry, witchcraft, astrology and the magic bough. It is no exaggeration that the magic bough (mistletoe) is demonstrating a remarkable reincarnation as Iscador, the most popular "unproven" remedy for the treatment of advanced cancer.

Literature and Theatre

The study of literature and theatre might have three important roles in the education of medical undergraduates –rebuilding medical idealism, deflating medical pomposity and providing us with a window into personal suffering.

It distressed me recently to learn that none of my of undergraduates at University College had read Axel Munthe's "The Story of San Michele" or A.J. Cronin's "The Citadel". For my generation of medical students these wonderful stories fuelled our idealism and there was no sense of shame in admitting at the interview for medical School entrance, that you wished to become a doctor out of idealism and a wish to serve humanity.

In contrast, the inhumane pompous and arrogant doctor who inevitably gets his comeuppance has been beautifully satirized in the works of Voltaire or George Bernard Shaw. I would like to recommend that all medical students read the preface to "Doctors Dilemma" as well as the play itself. The Sir Ralph Bloomfield Bonnington satirized by Shaw, still exists amongst the higher echelons of the medical establishment, but sadly we also see these attitudes amongst young doctors who know all about molecular biology on the one hand or managing a fund-holding practice on the other, but little about the feelings of the patient in the middle! Perhaps one of the best lessons in medical humility is to study the history of our subject and recognize that most of our added years and reduction in infant mortality has nothing to do with medicine but all to do with improvements in public health and the relief of poverty [13]. It was as much a result of the righteous indignation of idealistic politicians after reading the 19th C novels of Charles Dickens, as anything achieved by doctors in that time, that contributed to improvements in the welfare of infants and young children. [14] This same sense of righteous indignation should be experienced by medical students reading some the wonderful contemporary novels emerging from the Indian sub-continent or by first-hand experience doing electives in the developing world, getting out into the slums instead of spending time on Pataya beach. This recognition of the impact of social injustice on health will then educate the undergraduate in the true meaning of the ethics of distributive justice, health economics and the inevitability of rationing. It is the politician's right and responsibility to decide on what proportion of the gross National product should be allocated to welfare, housing or medicine. It is then left to the medical establishment to apportion their share of the cake to public health measures, primary health care or high technology medicine in the acute sector. The allocation of scarce resources within a just and humane Society, demands the recognition that our most precious resource is skilled manpower, and the more of this that is say allocated to organ transplantation, the less will be available for the not so glamorous pursuits such as the care of the elderly, the chronically infirm or the mentally ill.

Literature and the theatre also provide us with a window on personal suffering. We often talk about empathizing with our patients but this is a meaningless cliché without a genuine understanding of the fears and suffering of our patients. A pre-requisite for sensitive doctoring demands good communication skills that is dependent on genuine empathy, and the gift of listening. We should also exploit our patient's natural gift for story telling. We should teach our students patience in listening to the anecdotes of old soldiers and old sailors who were provided with free tobacco during the Second World War and then been admitted with ischaemia of their lower limbs to our modern high-tech hospitals. Students should respect the gift of story telling and not be confined to the straight jacket of the conventional history (patient complains of – history presenting complaint – past medical history etc). Taken to extreme, an individuals' experience of disease and suffering linked with a lyrical gift of poetry, literature and the transcendental can produce the most beautiful and moving prose [15]. For example Julia Rose, one of the most promising philosophers of our age, had her life cut short by cancer and published a book shortly before her diagnosis entitled "Loves Work" [16]. It is extremely moving to read this passage with the knowledge of what was awaiting her. "I would like to pass unnoticed which is why I hope that I am not deprived of old age, I aspire to a Miss Marple persona, to be exactly as I am, decrepit nature, yet super-nature in one, equally alert on the damp ground and in the turbulent air. Perhaps I don't have to wait for old age for that invisible trespass and pedestrian tread; insensible of mortality and desperately mortal".

When proposing literature, theatre and poetry as a component of the study of medicine, we have a powerful ally in the Lancet. This has been an important feature in the back pages of recent issues. I have little doubt therefore that we can persuade the Editor, to promote our cause through the most influential medical Journal in the UK, having recently published his proposal for a core canon of medical literature on 22nd March 1997 [17]

The History and Execution of Fine Art

Doctors, in addition to being interested in the history of art, are often gifted amateurs, and this trait is seen commonly amongst surgeons of the highest rank. For them art can be a therapy releasing them from the frustrations, tensions and anxieties of their day to day work by exercising the other half of the brain. But it is at this point that we stray into the territory of art as therapy, which is not strictly our remit. Yet my experience in being an advocate for art therapy in my years as Professor at the Royal Marsden Hospital, exposed me to the intense imagery provided by even the least gifted patient, providing them with a catharsis and us with an insight or a window into their suffering and fear. In many ways this is analogous to the role of literature but in this example all patients are able to express themselves even with the most naïve of images. Few however are sufficiently gifted to express themselves in writing.

Some time in 1990, shortly after I was appointed Professor of Surgery at the Royal Marsden Hospital, I was making a solitary ward round, checking on the welfare of my breast cancer patients, when I came upon an unfamiliar woman handing out pots of paint to a patient recovering from my surgical assault. Assuming she was an occupational therapist and wanting to make my presence felt, I engaged her in conversation. Within five minutes of talking to Camilla Connell, I was totally won over to the concept of art therapy for patients with cancer. Since that day, a warm relationship has developed between us, based on mutual respect and understanding for the contributions we can each make to patients recovering from cancer surgery, or for that matter, any other life-threatening disorder.

My interest and enthusiasm can be described at two levels. First, there is an uncanny thematic similarity running through the works of many of these patients who face serious disease. It is as if the experience of cancer stimulates some deeply hidden communal memory to evoke the symbolism of life and death, fear and hope. The tree, for example, is a recurring theme in these works of art, one that can be traced back through many cultures to the original *etz chaim* (tree of life) of the Old Testament.

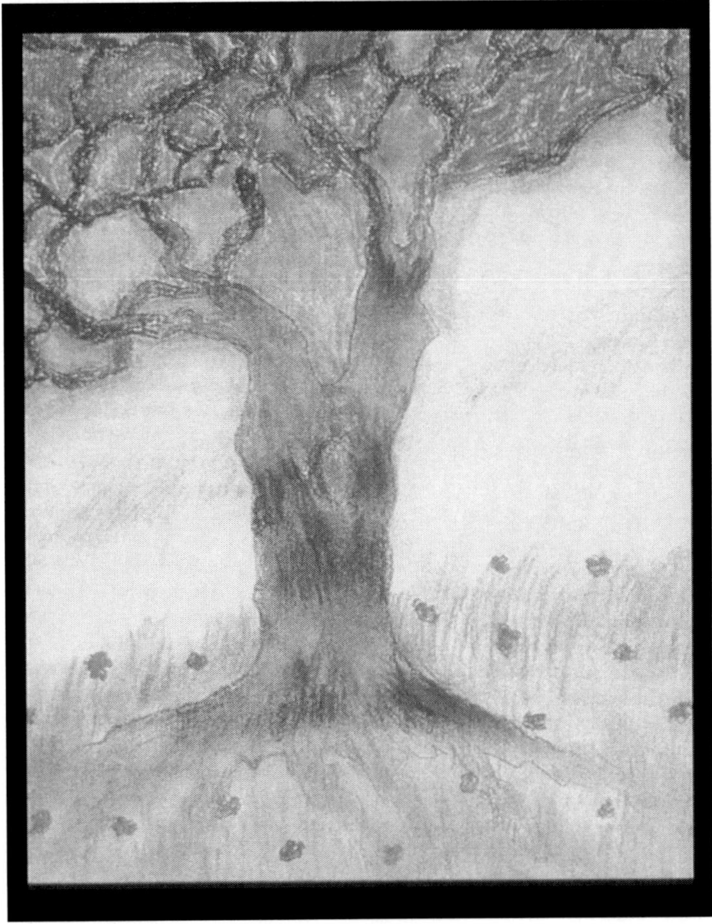

The tree of life.

At an individual level, what I have found so moving is the obvious cathartic value of using art to express hidden fears, the progression of the imagery from fear to hope as a sign of recovery and sadly, in the reverse direction, as a sign of deterioration. There is no doubt that art is a powerful medium for self-expression for frightened patients who do not have the words or the will to express themselves verbally.

Many patients have hidden talents, yet even in the absence of conventional artistic skill some of the, almost childlike and naïve, pictures are enormously expressive and deeply moving to the observer. I believe that art therapy is a unique vehicle for allowing patients with cancer to express hidden emotions and thus, to some extent, provide their own psychotherapy.

As a practical expression of my enthusiasm and support, I helped Camilla organize an exhibition of the patients' art, which was shown first at the Royal Marsden Hospital and then continued as a peripatetic exhibition around medical centres in the UK. I also used my authority to help raise funding for a second part-time art therapist to work at the Sutton branch of our Institution.

Whilst this was going on, the Marsden, like other cancer centres in London was facing closure as a result of the Tomlinson Report on the future of London hospital services. As Professor of Surgery and Director of Clinical Research, I was placed in the front line of the battle to save the hospital. This was also at a time when planning blight led to the early retirement of one of my Consultant colleagues and departure of another for a different teaching hospital. I was left to run the department virtually single-handed.

The stress of this workload and our uncertain future were almost too much to bear. I placed myself at Camilla's mercy to provide art therapy for my own struggle. I elected to undertake private tuition in portrait sculpture (which is her particular expertise). I learnt at first hand the benefits of self-expression through the medium of clay. The journey through a lifeless lump of material to a recognizable portrait of my daughter was sufficiently cathartic to help me cope with my struggles (I suspect that some of my fiercest attacks on the clay were surrogates for physical abuse of the bureaucrats who were trying to destroy the wonderful institution of the Royal Marsden Hospital.)

I therefore have both first and second-hand experience of the power of art therapy. I acknowledge that this is anecdotal evidence and as a clinical scientist, I would not accept art therapy on these merits alone – but I truly believe that it has a part to play in the management of the sick and the frightened, and that it is also a topic suitable for scientific evaluation using established instruments for the monitoring of patient's quality of life.

Good medicine is not only the practice of the science of the subject, but also the practice of the humanities of the subject. Central to the humanitarian practice of medicine is the development of good communication skills. Central to the development of good communication skills is the development of empathy. Strictly, empathy means trying to get inside the patient's head, to feel his or her fears and pain, a task that even the most empathetic of doctors can find extremely difficult. As far as I am concerned, art therapy is the most direct line into the patient's experience of illness, and I feel almost ashamed that I do not make use of it in the day-to-day practice of my own clinic. Perhaps there simply are not enough Camilla Connells to go round. If there were, I have little doubt that the drugs budget for the NHS would fall, as prescriptions for anxyolitics and anti-depressants would be replaced by the prescription of art therapy. [18]

The traditional link between art and medicine has been in the illustration of anatomy texts, and more recently the illustrations in textbooks, in particular for the techniques of complex surgical procedures. Perhaps the most famous textbook of anatomy of all time was published by Vesalius in the 16th Century and illustrated by Stephen van Calcar, one of Titian's ablest pupils.

Art is also a very powerful teaching medium. Wittingly, or unwittingly, great artists of the past have been skilled at illustrating the ravages of disease and deformity, and this has been a subject of fascination for artists and doctors alike in the last few decades. For example, Masaccio's Cripple illustrated in one of his Frescoes of the Brancacci chapel in Florence, or the goitre of Dante Gabriel Rossetti's favourite model. My personal favourite, is the inadvertent illustration of breast cancer in Rembrandt's moving painting of Bathsheba at her toilet in the Louvre Museum (p84). An Australian surgical resident, Peter Braithwaite, drew the dimple in her left breast to my attention. When I show this to medical students the impact is immediate. First of all it demonstrates the clinical signs of breast cancer, secondly it demonstrates that breast cancer is not a new disease and thirdly it illustrates the natural history of breast cancer where even without treatment patients can live for ten years.

Another direction that could be pursued is the way physical handicap might impact on artists and their creativity. A recent illustration both as a work of poetry and an illustration of art, concerned Monet's cataracts as described in the Lancet December 1996 [19]. One could argue whether the cataracts contributed to his creativity as suggested by the author of the piece, or in my opinion that the maturation of any artist with or without visual impairment can improve on creativity. The same enigma applies to El Greco's paintings with their astigmatic appearance. Historians of art, who argue that the visual defect contributed to El Greco's perception, have obviously overlooked the logical solecism of this interpretation. Renoir's rheumatoid arthritis meant that he had to paint with his brushes strapped to his wrist, and yet this if anything enhanced the quality of his work [20]. Aubrey Beardsley's fevered imagination was fuelled by his tuberculosis. There are many parallels to the poetry of John Keats who also died at a tragically young age from tuberculosis. It is also worth reading biographies of Aubrey Beardsley who frittered away the last couple of years of his life chasing miracle cures amongst the watering holes of Europe. Or better still Thomas Mann's "The Magic Mountain", that perfectly describes the atmosphere of a sanatorium in the Swiss Alps, where the comfortably off young wasted their youth in the futile pursuit of the "fresh air cure", the fashionable quackery of its day. [21] In fact the whole subject of creativity and disease has been covered in a beautiful short monograph by Professor Philip Sandbolm of Gotenberg University, Sweden: a delightful and accessible source of material for student projects. [22]

Somehow I've been able to convince the curriculum committee of my medical school that all of the above makes a suitable special study module (SSM) for a select group of our first year students. The high spot of my week now is Thursday afternoon that is spent with a dozen students who share my enthusiasm. Whether my self-indulgence does them any good is open to speculation, but a couple of hours a week spent in one of our National treasure houses of fine Art, is powerful medicine for the author!

Musical Performance and Appreciation

Exactly as with painting, music can be therapy for the doctor as well as the patient, either in its performance or in its appreciation. Many physicians are amateur musicians and no doubt enjoy a release from the tensions of being a doctor when performing. And to discuss music as therapy is once again outside our remit.

There is a fascinating linkage between the appreciation of music and of speech, and yet there are paradoxical relationships between aphasia and amusia. Oliver Sacks, a physician with the gift of an accomplished writer, describes many such examples from his experience, and in particular in his delightful book of short anecdotes "The Man Who Mistook His Wife For A Hat". [23] There are patients with severe mental or neurological disabilities who are capable of appreciating or performing music at the highest levels. As with art, the great composers have suffered disease that has affected their physical and mental well being, which inevitably has had an influence on their creativity. Once again this subject is covered in Philip Sandblom's monograph or more recently in Anton Neumayr's book, "Music and Medicine" (24) In parallel with my discussion about artists and their perception, one could discuss the impact of Beethoven's deafness and the creativity of his latter years alongside Monet's cataracts and his perception of the House of Commons at twilight.

At this point I would like to briefly mention opera. The opera is a remarkable amalgam of theatre, design, spectacle and music, but inevitably one has to ask the awkward question "do the death scenes of Mimi and Violetta in La Boheme and La Traviata add pathos or bathos to terminal tuberculosis?" This delicate balance depends heavily on the sensitivity of the Director that is another aspect of the performing arts. The Doctor as Director has a fine tradition and of course the leading contemporary exponent is Dr Jonathan Miller.

How Can We Make This All Happen?

To introduce the Arts and Humanities into the undergraduate curriculum we need the political will of the medical establishment at the highest level, adequate funding and space within an overcrowded curriculum. Of these three the first has been achieved unequivocally. As far as the second is concerned we will need major funding that might be available through the Lottery Commission or the Millennium Fund. Perhaps most difficult of all will be finding adequate space within a curriculum which is already considered over-crowded and which is undergoing an upheaval with the implementation of the new GMC recommendations. Yet at the same time the recommendations on the undergraduate medical education "Tomorrow's Doctors", published by the General Medical Council has given us the green light. For example under Section 29 page 10, you can read the following paragraph... "As medical research advances it will inevitably become increasingly dependent on the ideas and techniques of other disciplines. On mathematics and physics in the elucidation of complex biomedical phenomena on the social sciences and philosophy in confronting the wide range of cultural, environmental and ethical issues that will increasingly impinge on the problems of health. It is hoped that the student of tomorrow may be drawn towards some of these other disciplines and that opportunities to study for example a language or to undertake a project related to literature or the history of medicine, may be offered". [25]

Whatever the sub-specialty, any under-graduate teaching Firm is the ideal setting for the teaching of narrative and through narrative enhance the communication skills of the students, their capacity to listen and their capacity to empathize. Tricia Greenhalgh and Brian Hurwitz published a very important paper in the British Medical Journal last year, describing the justification for the study of narrative [26]. I have personally taken the subject one step forward by actively encouraging my students to collect the patient's narrative and write them up as a piece of literature, encouraging them to draw on all their skills and enthusiasms that antedated their entry into Medical School and which like any other talent atrophies with disuse. To further help and encourage them in this endeavour I insist that they read literature outside their medical textbooks and promise them that this will become a labour of love. Faith McLellan and Ann Hudson-Jones, both from the Institute of Medical Humanities at the University of Texas, Galveston, have written much on the importance of the study of literature by medical students and Ann Hudson-Jones has described an evolving canon of literature that will enhance the student's understanding of the experience of ill health.

Conclusion

One Sunday evening in December last year, my wife and I went to the Barbican to listen to Verdi's Requiem. The interior architecture and the gold ochre of the wood produced an immediate sense of peace and tranquility. The music and poetry of the piece eloquently describe the fear of death, the terror of the Day of Judgment, yet also the optimism and faith in a rebirth of the spirit. For example, the verses 2-5 of the sequence with the extraordinary trumpeting from the brass section that makes the hair on the back of your scalp stand on end, says it all "*quantus tremor est futures*.... How great a terror there will be when the Judge shall come, he who shall examine all things strictly – the trumpet spreading its wondrous sound to the tombs of the whole world, will bring everyone before the throne. Death and nature shall be dumbfounded when creation rises again to answer its Judge". Finally in the last section, *Agnus Dei* the words of solace, and the change from the minor to the major key, allow you to leave the auditorium with your despair replaced by euphoria and optimism. This could be looked upon as a version of spiritual healing for the terminally ill or at a more mundane level, anxiolytic therapy on a Sunday evening for doctors having to face the stresses of the week ahead. Either way, Verdi has enriched the life of many, including myself. I would like to think my patients find me a more amiable and tolerant doctor on a Monday morning than I would otherwise be without his help.

References

[1] Not a slippery slope or sudden subversion: German medicine and National Socialism in 1933 Hanauske-Abel, H.M. *Brit.Med.J.* 1996;313:1453-1463.

[2] Humanities in Medicine Beyond the Millenium, Ed. Robin Philipp,Michael Baum,Andrew Mawson and Sir Kenneth Calman Nuffield Trust Series No.10 ,London 1998.

[3] The Two Cultures and the Scientific Revolution, *The Rede Lecture* 1959, Cambridge University Press.

[4] The Quest for pure truth. Melvyn Bragg; Independent on Sunday 8th March 1998.

[5] Why Arts courses for medical curricula? Calman K. and Downie R. *Lancet* 1996; 347: 1499-1500.

[6] The Logic of Scientific discovery, Popper K. R. Hutchinson: London 1968.

[7] The Structure of Scientific Revolutions, T.S. Kuhn, Chicago; University of Chicago Press, 1970.

[8] Zen and the Art of Motorcycle maintenance , Robert M. Pirsig, Bantam Books , Toronto/New York/ London , 15th printing 1976.

[9] Janus: a summing up, Arthur Koestler, Picador London , 1979.

[10] Quack cancer cures or scientific remedies, Baum M. J. R. *Soc Med* 1996;89:543-547.

[11] Principles of Biomedical ethics, 3rd edition 1989. Beauchamp T and Childress J, Oxford University Press, New York, Oxford.

[12] Religion, spirituality, and medicine Sloan RP , Bagiella E , Powell T, *The Lancet* 1999;353: 664-667.

[13] High Technology Medicine: Benefits and burdens. Jennett, B. Oxford, Oxford University Press, 1986

[14] The greatest benefit to mankind, Roy Porter , Harper Collins London, 1997.

[15] Why Literature and Medicine? McLellan M F and Hudson Jones A. *The Lancet* 1996 ;348: 109-111.

[16] Love's Work, Gillian Rose, Schocken Books, New York 1996.

[17] A manifesto for reading medicine Horton R. *The Lancet* 1997; 349:872-874.

[18] The Arts of healing Friedrich, M. J. *Journal of the American Medical Association* 1999: 281: 1770-1781.

[19] Literature and medicine: the patient, the physician, and the poem. McLellan MF. *The Lancet* 1996;348: 1640-1641.

[20] How Renoir coped with rheumatoid arthritis. Boonen A ,van de Rest J, Dequeker J ,van der Linden S. *The Lancet* 1997 ; 315:1704-1708.

[21] The magic mountain. Thomas Mann, First published 1924, Recent English translation by H.T. Lowe-Porter, Vintage, London 1999.

[22] Creativity and disease, Philip Sandblom George F. Stickley and Co. Philadelphia, 4th edition 1987.

[23] The man who mistook his wife for a hat. Oliver Sacks, Picador London 1986.

[24] Music and Medicine, Anton Neumayr Medi-Ed press; Bloomington, Illinois, 1995.

[25] General Medical Council education committee. *Tomorrow's doctors*: GMC, 1993.

[26] Narrative based medicine; Why study Narrative? Trisha Greenalgh and Brian Hurwitz, *Brit Med J* ;318: 48-50, 2000.

Chapter 9

Evidence Based Art?

(J R Soc Med 2001 94: 306-307)

"A recent meta-analysis of randomised controlled trials of the presence or absence of paintings in wards has demonstrated some far-reaching results. It is estimated that looking at paintings, whilst confined to bed lowers the blood pressure by a mean value of 5mms of mercury whilst raising a sense of wellbeing by an average of seven QUALIS (Quality adjusted laughter indices). These results, if extrapolated across the UK could save £40,000,000 in the prescription of beta-blockers and £120,000,000 in the prescription of anti-depressants. A government spokesman responded to these observations by promising to recruit 120 artists in residence over the next ten years."

Of course I made that all up and yet it is not all that far fetched, particularly if the bean counters have their way. These thoughts occurred to me on a journey back from Exeter earlier this year where I had attended an all day conference to launch the evaluation of the Exeter healthcare arts project.

The Royal Devon & Exeter Hospital is a low rise, modern development built around a series of courtyards. The Courtyards contain pieces of modern sculpture set amongst peaceful gardens both Zen and non-Zen in their inspiration. The walls are richly covered with contemporary art and photography. They are magnificent tapestries and mosaics in the entrance hall and if you will forgive the expression, a chapel to die for! Mr Peter Senior, the Director for the Arts for Health Dept at the Manchester Metropolitan

University had been commissioned to audit and evaluate this extraordinary collection and the launch of this evaluation was the excuse for my visit.

As a scientific exercise it lacked something of the rigour of the randomised controlled trial or the case controlled study central to the practice of evidence based medicine. Essentially staff and patients were asked whether they liked the environment and whether or not being surrounded by beautiful things enriched their life.

In the passionate debate that followed, it was possible to witness the audience polarised into the strict scientific empiricists and the "fuzzy logic" experientialists. As someone steeped in the traditions of the randomised controlled trials and an advocate of the scientific process my initial sympathies swung behind the scientific empirical wing of the audience. I could easily imagine how one could design an experiment whereby patients requiring radiotherapy were randomised into one of four bunkers in a 2 x 2 factorial design. One bunker would have its grey walls unadorned. Another bunker would be filled with Mozart's music, a third bunker would have its walls covered in murals by Raoul Dufy and the fourth bunker would have both the art and the music. Outcome measures would include quality of life as measured by the hospital anxiety depression score (HADS) and objective measures such as natural killer cell count and relapse free survival. However, more mature consideration on the train back home convinced me that these ideas were utterly absurd; an abuse of not only the arts culture, but also the science culture as well.

Hospital wards and corridors are public places. They are also the temporary homes of our medical charges. Which public places are denied their fill of works of art and how many philistines are there whose homes are not filled with pictures or throb to the beat of the base guitar? The value of art and music are givens within our culture and the life enhancing value of fine art is common experience to us all. Indeed it is highly likely that the sense of wellbeing when contemplating a work of art is associated with the lowering of blood pressure and other beneficial physiological changes - a subject well worthy of research. But these are "side effects" and only surrogates for the real outcome.

Coming back to the Chapel at Exeter, the architectural shape of the space for prayer, the colour scheme on the walls, the maple furniture and the paintings and tapestries adorning the walls generated a sense of calm similar to that, which I experience in the Tate Modern Gallery in the room devoted to the large abstract paintings of Mark Rothko. I assure you, this **wasn't** measured on the environmental calming index (ECI) In other words whether a practising

Christian or a secularist, time spent sitting in the chapel makes you feel good. It then occurred to me that it has been accepted for more than 200 years that a Chapel is an integral component of a hospital, yet I have never heard a voice that demands a randomised controlled trial of chapels in hospitals. Once again these are givens within our Society.

Come to think of it, in my own planning blighted hospital, The Middlesex of Mortimer Street, there are only two sanctuaries that are pleasing to the eye and pleasing to the spirit.

The entrance hall still proudly displays the large paintings by Frederick Caylay Robinson (1864-1926) showing the nurses descending and ascending for their breakfast - an allegory for the angels of healing, flanked on each side by allegorical paintings of the three ages of man and the resurrection of the fallen from the 1st World War.

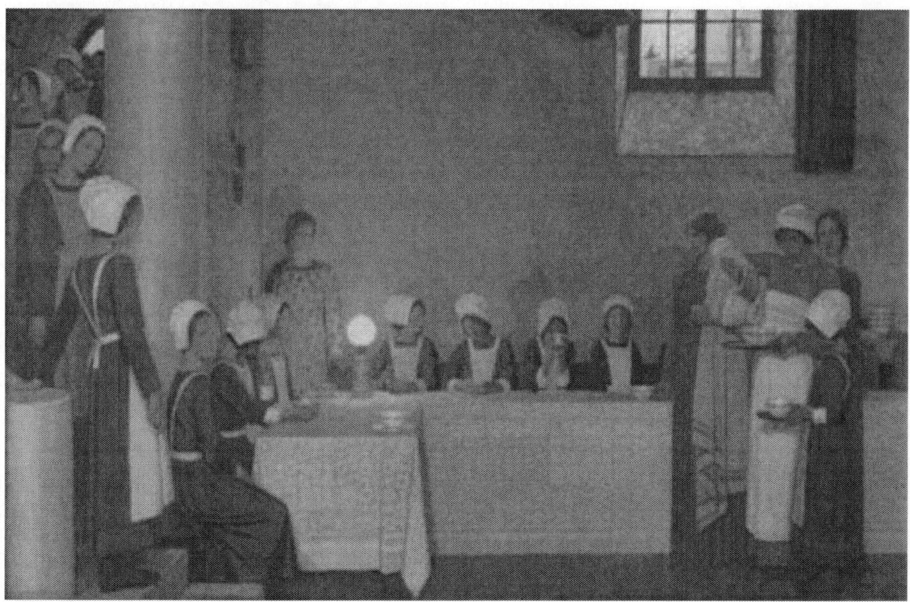

Acts of Mercy, Cayley-Robinson.

Even amongst the hustle and bustle and the visual pollution of a decaying NHS hospital, these pictures exert their calming influence on me. The other sanctuary is the pretty little Victorian chapel that I pass most days with an envious glance at those whose time and creed allow a moment or two of contemplation.

The humanities and the sciences have their equal roles in the practice of medicine. Each should be respected by the other and without this mutual respect we are all diminished. To me the notion of evidence-based art is as absurd as a French Impressionist school of Science.

Chapter 10

Book Review for JRSM

The Healing Environment: Without and within
Edited by Deborah Kirklin & Ruth Richardson

Introduction

Book reviews can take on a life of their own and often serve as a platform for the reviewer to parade their political viewpoint or pedal their prejudices. I elect at the indulgence of Robin Fox, editor of JRSM, to use this platform to express my concern that the medical humanities movement, of which I am a fully paid up member [1], is in danger of losing its way.

The editor of this journal challenged me to write this book review as a follow up to a mischievous paper I published in the JRSM a couple of years ago with the title "Evidence based Art" [2]. I quote from it to give you a flavour of my thinking.

"The humanities and the sciences have their equal roles in the practice of medicine. Each should be respected by the other and without this mutual respect we are all diminished. To me the notion of evidence based art is as absurd as a French Impressionist school of Science."

To begin with I thought this book would reinforce my prejudice as Prof. Carol Black, PRCP states in her preface that the Arts and Humanities are of *"immeasurable importance"*. This I took literally as meaning not lending itself to measurement.

Yet, Lara Dose, Director of the National Network of the Arts in Health, in her excellent forward states *" Money will only be forthcoming once the evidence of the efficacy of arts-based health interventions is available. Whilst many working within this field view the results of their work as self-evident, it is now clear that funders.... do require a persuasive evidence base before they will commit any money"*

What a depressing thought that the bean counters require evidence that beauty is good for you.

Fine. I can accept the need for well-designed experiments for the therapeutic claims of art or poetry therapy before we start employing poets and painters in residence but surely not for the justification of a beautiful and quiet environment in which we care for the sick or within which we have to work as health care providers.

Hospital wards and corridors are public places. They are also the temporary homes of our medical charges. Which public places are denied natural light, an interesting view or at least walls punctuated with works of art? How many philistines are there whose homes are completely empty of pictures or whose walls are painted an institutional cream colour? The value of art, literature, poetry and music are givens within our culture and their life enhancing value is common experience to us all. Indeed it is highly likely that the sense of well-being when contemplating a work of art, reading poetry or listening to a symphony are associated with the lowering of blood pressure, raising the lymphocyte count, endorphin release and other beneficial physiological changes, subjects well worthy of research, but these are "side effects", surrogates for the real outcome.

In fact I was nearly half way through this book before I fully understood the significance of its title. I approached it in all innocence assuming we would be learning about the importance of architecture and Art in providing the right environment for clinical staff to carry out their work of healing. As it turns out about half the book is devoted to the patients "internal environment" not defined in physiological terms but in a metaphysical manner somewhere in the realms of "spirit" or "soul". Perhaps these are the real outcomes I refer to above rather than the physiological "*milieu interieur*". In spite of my natural sympathy I was left extremely irritated by the chapter by John Fox, a certified poetry therapist, who implied that failure to share these metaphysical models of the inner self implied doctors were spiritually stunted and not sufficiently soulful. Maybe we are, however it is a grave error of judgment for the practitioners in the field of medical humanities to adopt the spiritual and moral high ground only to alienate those working at the coalface. Yes, many working environments are brutal and yes, many clinical practices appear inhumane. Yet we must start from the default position that *all* medical practitioners are decent and cultured folk and root cause analysis will show the fault lies with our education and a health service that understands the price of everything and the value of nothing!

What we end up with are 12 essays, mostly very well written, readable and often deeply moving which are only tenuously linked. About half address the outer environment and the others consider the spiritual dimension. About half attempt to produce experimental evidence to support their claims whilst the others are mercifully free of attempts to quantify the soul. Where experimental evidence is presented it is almost impossible to evaluate either because the methodology is inadequately described or is seriously flawed.

This is amply illustrated by two chapters linked to the Chelsea and Westminster (C&M) Hospital Arts group. In the first, "Integrating the arts into health care: can we affect the clinical outcomes?" Rosalina Staricoff & Susan Loppert, state "*The need for a rigorous evaluation of the effects of the arts in health care is widely recognized and the Chelsea & Westminster provides an ideal setting for such an evaluation process*". As far as the latter assertion is concerned I couldn't disagree more strongly. The C&M is a one off show place. It was built way over budget and the expense of destabilizing health care in West London and as I learnt to the cost of my personal health, when the future of the Royal Marsden Hospital was placed in jeopardy. The C&M bears as much relationship to the average NHS hospital as St Peter's Cathedral in Rome does to your parish church! Let those who can, enjoy its interior and fine commissioned works of art, but it is smug to claim that the C&M is an exemplar of what might be achieved in Slagthorpe under Lyme, District General Hospital. Furthermore that wonderful work by Allen Jones of the acrobat hanging in the atrium, the largest indoor sculpture in the UK, was put in without an evidence base that it is good for the health of the patients. Yet I cannot conceive of an experiment nor would I endorse one, to falsify that hypothesis.

That aside, let us consider the rigor of their evaluation of art and music. For the most part, the qualitative responses of the public were in favour of beauty: blindingly self-evident. The experimental studies were insufficiently described in detail from a referee's point of view but can be judged indirectly by these statements. *"The small size of the sample made it impossible to detect significant differences", "This was a pilot study with 34 patients in the control group and 54 in the study group...........results suggest a tendency to lower levels of blood pressure......"*. I suggest that in future they employ statisticians at the start of a project for power calculations and randomization techniques. The same criticisms can apply in the linked chapter by Jane Duncan attempting to evaluate the impact of a gorgeous set of murals and ceiling paintings on a blank and forbidding hydrotherapy unit. She clearly admits that the quantitative results were disappointing and attempts to rationalize them away. Jane, as one artist to another; take my word on this, your work is beautiful and even in reproduction in a book, enhanced my life.

As this book is replete with delightful and illuminating anecdotes, I feel I have the right to offer one of my own that at the same time illustrates the strengths and the weaknesses of this collection of essays.

One Friday evening, a few days before Christmas last year, Annie, my lovely and feisty 96-year-old *Geordie*[1] mother in law, needed to be admitted as an emergency to our local hospital with acute viral pneumonia. Up until then she had "all her marbles" and played a mean game of contract bridge. The ambulance arrived promptly and she was delivered to the subterranean A&E department. After a reasonable delay she was medically evaluated and admission to the ward was arranged. For the next six hours she lay on a trolley in a featureless and windowless room getting more and more disorientated and frightened in spite of the presence of my wife and I. At last she was admitted to the receiving ward another blank featureless room with four beds. In one corner was a comatose and dying woman with a grieving family at the bedside. In the next corner was a demented old lady screaming non stop abuse and exposing herself to all comers.

And finally, in the adjacent bed next to Annie, was a middle-eastern lady, surrounded by an affectionate but boisterous family who came and went in droves treating the place like a souk! All of these patients had their own needs for "healing environments" yet all were denied them. The Arabic lady deserved to be embraced by her loving family, but not at the price of peace and quiet for Annie to recover. The demented old lady was denied the dignity of succumbing to or recovering from whatever had precipitated the acute episode whilst her family should have been spared the mortification of her public behaviour. Finally the family of a dying woman should have been allowed their vigil in peace. And for everyone's sake flowers, potted plants, walls of warm and friendly colours and pictures filling in the gaps would have helped to lift the grim pall that hung over the ward. As a Christmas miracle and thanks to the devoted care of an understaffed ward of nurses (not an Anglo-Saxon face among them by the way), she returned to her cosy little warden-protected accommodation, on New Year's Day.

This now leads me to what I believe is the best chapter in the book, "Healing by design: feeling better", by John Wells-Thorpe. In this he describes the exploitation of a "natural experiment" afforded by a "before and after" study of patients in two hospitals, an orthopaedic unit in Poole and a mental health unit in Brighton, being translocated to modern architect designed facilities round about the same time. The new facilities were designed in an attempt to centre the activity around the patients needs whereas the old units are described as places where *" the hospital bed can be perceived by patients not as a safe haven, but rather as a medium of containment which renders the patient as a passive object of clinician's activity"*. The outcomes of this study were very impressive yet in a way confirming the obvious that light, colour and a view from the window helped recovery, yet the one unpredicted outcome considered far and away the most important by the consumers was the manner in which the new environments *enabled or inhibited privacy or sociability*.

By the way I forgot to mention-my local hospital is the Royal Free in Hampstead, home of the centre housing the editors of this publication. Perhaps before going any further with the work on art appreciation, creative writing and poetry therapy, for healing the soul, they might like to do a ward round and do something about the gruesome external environment of their wards that debilitates the spirit of patient, staff and family. The Royal Free sets the challenge more than The Chelsea and Westminster, because this unlovely structure has none of the inbuilt advantages of the latter and thus is more relevant to the NHS as a whole.

Conclusion

I believe that Art, music and the humanities in general enhance our daily lives and make sense of our very existence. As such they should not be denied us when we are sick and dying. Furthermore they should not be subject to audit.

At the same time I believe that any activity with "therapy" in its title should be subject to critical evaluation to avoid diversion of scarce resources without sound evidence. There is only one standard of evaluation and that involves careful consideration of outcome measurement and experimental design. There can be no compromise even if "the therapy" is art based. Failure to do this will relegate these subjects to the realm of "alternative" medicine.

Finally I believe that these subjects should be integrated into the undergraduate and post graduate curricula providing they are monitored as with all other educational interventions and not enjoying a privileged position as new clothes on an old emperor. [3]

References

[1] Teaching the humanities to medical students, Baum M, *Clinical Medicine,* 2002, 2; 246 -249.

[2] Evidence-based art? Baum M, J R. *Soc Med* 2001 94: 306-307.

[3] Monitoring the education revolution: The impact of new training programmes must be evaluated. Wass V, Richards T, Cantillon P, *BMJ,* 2003, 327;1362.

Chapter 11

The Art of Oncology: The Changing Faces of Breast Cancer Treatment

(Programme notes for IBCC 3, held in the Louvre, Paris 2009, sponsored by Sanfoni Aventis)

Rembrandt's Bathsheba

The Louvre, Paris, houses a large and beguiling masterpiece by Rembrandt, "Bathsheba at her toilet". Completed in 1655, the painting shows a naked Bathsheba looking wistfully into the middle distance left, whilst holding a letter in her right hand. Her attendant bathes her feet in a pool and the background is dark and ambiguous. Perhaps she has just learnt of her husband's death in battle as a result of King's David's treachery, leaving her free to join the long list of the royal concubines.

About 25 years ago, a young Australian research fellow, Peter Braithwaite, drew my attention to the dimple in the upper outer quadrant of Bathsheba's left breast. I had to agree with him, the model for this painting has the classical stigma of breast cancer, which I have confirmed on subsequent visits to the Louvre to see the painting in the flesh, so to speak. I encouraged him to research the history of the painting and its model. His work on this ultimately appeared in print, since when Bathsheba has become an icon of the breast cancer movement. [1] In short, the model was Hendrekje Stoffels who doubled up as mistress and housekeeper for Rembrandt. She was in her thirties when the picture was completed and died eight years later. [2] Her mode of dying was characteristic of breast cancer with secondaries to the liver. There is no record of her being treated, but in any case treatment in those days was a futile hocus-pocus based on the doctrines of Aristotle and Galen, yet she lived eight years after the clinically obvious disease became apparent, unknowingly portrayed in the painting.

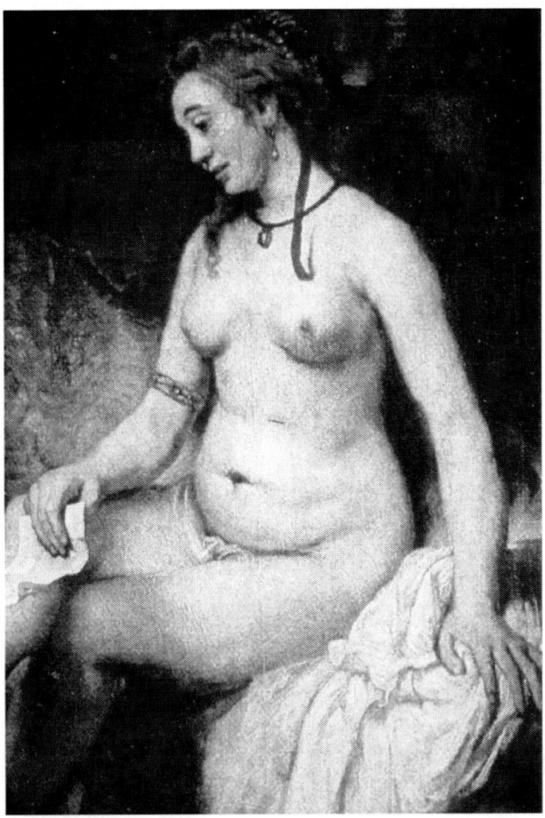

Bathsheba at her toilet.

For me, this is probably the best-attested chance illustration of breast cancer in the history of fine art. However, like many subjects in the field of art history, Bathsheba has stimulated its own share of debate and diverging opinions. Even the identity of the model has been brought into question. Based on X -rays of the painting showing that the position of the head was "altered", a Russian scholar, Dymarski, has suggested that Hendrikje's head may have been painted on someone else's body. [3]. Using these X-ray "findings", R.G. Bourne, puts forth alternate "diagnoses" depending upon to whom the model's body belonged. Given the eight years she lived from the time of the painting until her death, if the body was Hendrekje's, Bourne makes the case for tuberculous mastitis with axillary nodal involvement. If the body belonged to some other unknown model, he feels that breast cancer is the more likely explanation for what we see on the canvas.

Variety in interpretation is the spice of life, and we delight in the opportunity to comment and reflect on what the artist has masterfully portrayed. In the absence of more precise historical records, let alone pathological reports, Bathsheba may well be fostering debate and discussion for some time to come.

References

[1] Braithwaite PA and Shugg D. Rembrandt's Bathsheba: the dark shadow of the left breast. *Annals of the Royal College of Surgeons* 1983; 65: 337-339.

[2] Jessica B. Mandell, Bathsheba's breast Women, cancer & history J Clin Invest. 2005 June 1; 115(6): 1397.

[3] R. G. Bourne, Did Rembrandt'sS Bahtsheba Really Have Breast Cancer? *Aust. N.Z. J. Surg.* (2000) **70**, 231–232

Rafael's La Fornarina

A paper entitled "The portrait of breast cancer and Raphael's La Fornarina" by Espinal, published in the Lancet in December 2002 [1], claimed that Raphael's last painting of his mistress *La Fornarina,* was pointing to a cancer in her left breast. The author sited her position, the size and shape of the left breast and arm, an irregularity near the left axilla and skin colour discolouration as evidence for breast cancer. I have arrived at a different conclusion; that La Fornarina ***does not*** have breast cancer.

As many radiotherapists have learnt to their cost, the apex of the heart is deep to the left breast. Margherita, Raphael's model, is pointing to her heart as a token of her love for the artist. The hand or finger resting on the left breast is a classic pose from the times of antiquity much favoured during the Southern Renaissance. The "love band" inscribed with the name Raphael on the left upper arm provides further evidence. The closeness of their relationship is also supported by the evidence that La Fornarina's portrait was found in Raphael's studio after his death. [2,3]

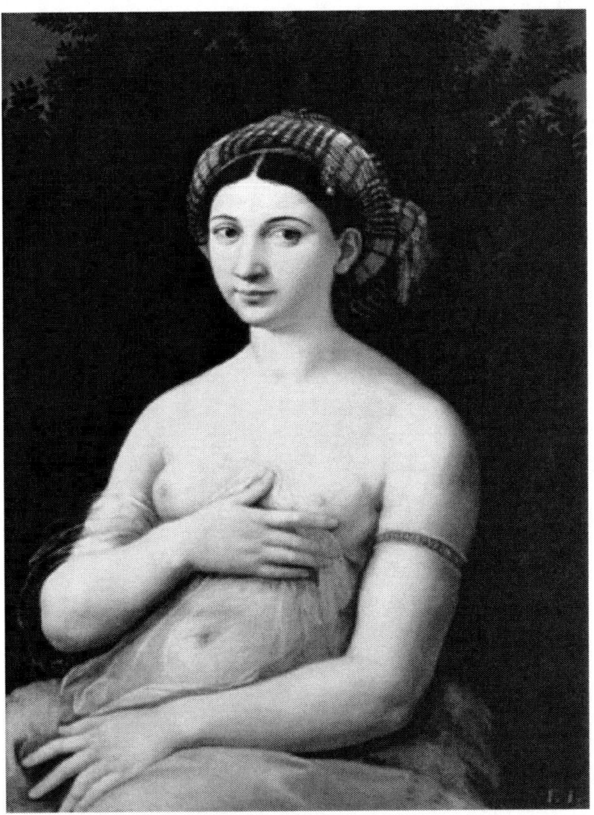

La Fornarina.

The author also asserts that a puckering of the breast just above the left index finger is evidence of a cancerous mass. However, a simple experiment will demonstrate that if a woman applies gentle pressure with the index finger, just below the left nipple, a linear dimple will appear. The author also sites nine hues colored black, taupe, umber, grey, purple, blue, cream, pink and brown as evidence for breast cancer related color changes. However, these are actually the standard colors and techniques used to depict gradations of shadow in 16th Century Italy [4,5]. Espinel also suggests that advanced carcinoma of the breast leads to blue discoloration of the skin. The available literature does not support this observation and in thirty plus years as a breast surgeon I've never personally observed a blue breast! Espinel goes onto suggest that the left breast is enlarged and that the left arm is abnormally swollen due to oedema and inflammation from the adjacent cancerous mass in the left breast. These statements are difficult to support as Margherita is turned a quarter away from the viewer introducing the possibility of parallax error when making estimations regarding size [6]. Indeed the right arm and right breast are not fully in view with the lateral mass of the right breast occluded by the overriding right arm. This conclusion also fails to recognize different body types, arm-body ratios and inter and intra-individual variations with women having different breast sizes and there may be a non-pathogenic size asymmetry between left and right breasts [7].

Why should art and history papers not be subjected to the same rigorous methods of evidence-based scholastic analysis?

References

[1] Espinel CH. The portrait of breast cancer and Raphael's La Fornarina. *The Lancet* 2002; 360: 2061-2063.

[2] Onori LM. La Fornarina. Biography of a painting. In: Nitti P, Restellini M and Sirinati C, Editors. *Raphael: grace and beauty*. Milan: Skira Editore 2001; pages 69–79.

[3] 3 Arasse D. The workshop of grace. In: Nitti P, Restellini M and Sirinati C, Editors. *Raphael: grace and beauty*. Milan: Skira Editore 2001; pages 57–68.

[4] Israel Zohar. Colours and techniques used to depict gradations of shadow in 16th Century Italy. Personal Communication 2003.

[5] Zohar I. Homage to Vermeer, Museum Panorama Mesdag, the Hague. London: Masters Group International Ltd. 1996.

[6] Kaminer MS, Dover JS and Arndt KA. Atlas of Cosmetic Surgery. Philadelphia: W.B. Saunders Company 2002.7. Epstein O, Perkin D, de Bono DP and Cookson J. Female Breasts and Genitalia. In: *Clinical Examination* 2nd edition, page 221.

Evelyn

This is a contemporary painting by a young English artist, Heath Rosselli.

When I first saw this arresting image I was captivated by the light of intelligence in the eyes, the beauty and self-confidence in the facial expression and sense of calm. It was a moment or two before I noticed that Evelyn had suffered a right mastectomy. I use this image in my lectures and as a frontispiece for a book and others have made the same comments. This tells me something about this women and women in general. Women are far more than the sum of the parts of their sexual identity.

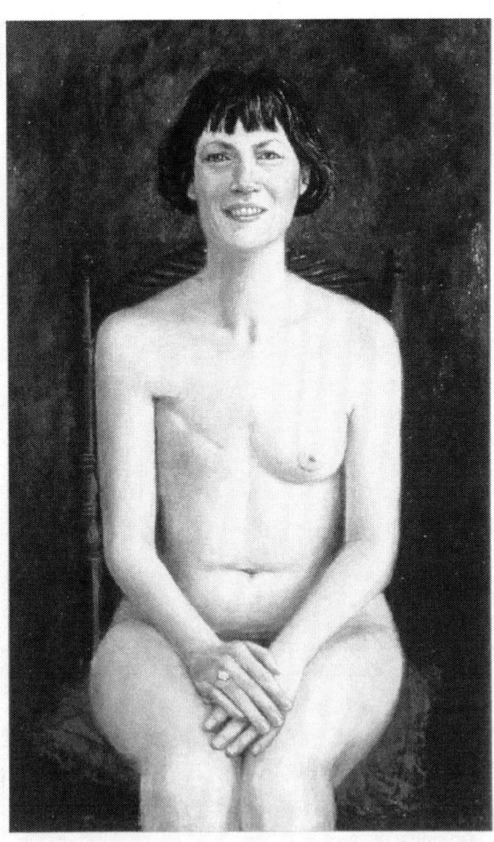

There is life after mastectomy. Portrait by Heath Rosselli, reproduced with kind permission from the artist.

Evelyn by Heath Rosselli.

Women have courage of a different sort to men. Men may win medals on the battlefield but there are no medals struck for women in bringing up the family whilst keeping the home fires burning. The majority of my patients face up to the diagnosis of breast cancer and its treatment with formidable bravery and often express sympathy with me for having to break the bad news! In addition they often show more concern for their husbands and children than themselves.

Many years ago I carried out some research with Lesley Fallowfield on the psycho-social and psycho-sexual consequences of mastectomy within a randomized controlled trial of mastectomy and breast conserving surgery. [1, 2] We were amazed to discover how well women cope with mastectomy even in the days before reconstruction was a default option.

Clinicians such as us should consider it a rare privilege that so many women have trusted their lives and their bodies to our medical and surgical skills. We therefore carry the moral obligation for self-improvement by attending conferences such as these.

References

[1] Fallowfield LJ, Baum M, Maguire GP. Effects of breast conservation on psychological morbidity associated with diagnosis and treatment of early breast cancer. *Br Med J* 1986;293:1331-1334.

[2] Fallowfield LJ, Hall A, Macquire GP, Baum M. Psychological outcomes in women with early breast cancer. *Br Med J* 1990;301:1394.

Ruben's the Three Graces

I must start off with a confession. Ruben's is not one of my favorite painters. His histrionic poses and over populated huge paintings does nothing for me and I'm almost ashamed to say that his idealized vision of female beauty it not shared by me. Give me Botticelli's favorite model, Simonetta Vespucci (she of the birth of Venus and Primavera) any day. "The three Graces" was painted around 1636. The model for this figure is Ruben's second wife Helena Fourment. Rubens married her (1614–1673) on December 6, 1630, when he was fifty-three and she was sixteen. Helena became the model and the inspiration for many paintings by Rubens dating from the 1630s, particularly those dealing with themes of ideal beauty or love. Simon Schama in his magnum opus "Rembrandt's eyes" pays homage to the beauty of Helena and describes how many of Ruben's portraits of his young wife suggested "she submitted herself to his hungry gaze" [1]

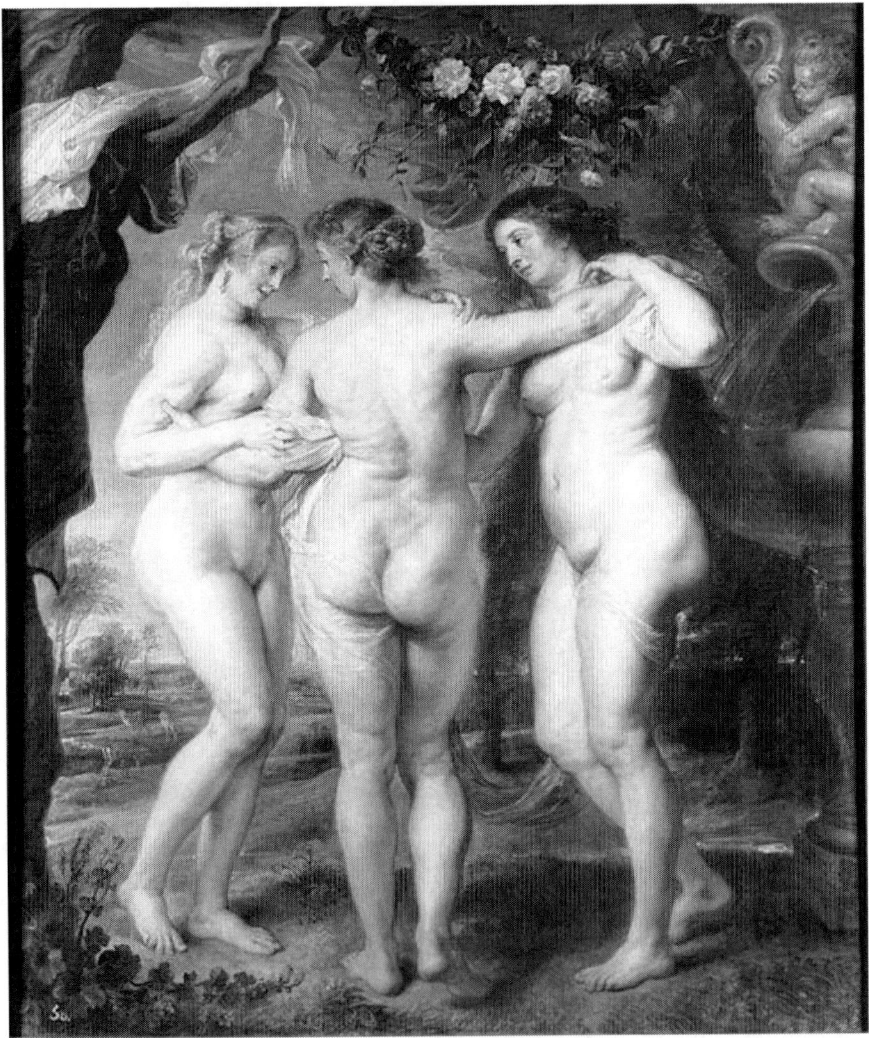

Rubens "The three Graces.

One painting in particular "Het Pelsken" showing Helena half draped in a fur skin at the age of 24 with opulent breasts and erect nipples proudly on display, was judged indecent by the model herself and kept hidden after Ruben's death. Helena was left with five children and a huge fortune and died at the age of 59. I can find no description or speculation about her cause of death although the age itself might suggest breast cancer as a candidate. But to return to the painting in question; indeed there is a deep crease in the upper outer of her left breast but to my eye that is not like the dimple seen in Hendrekje Stoffels' left breast. Natural skin creases like this are common in well-covered women and a gift for the surgeon who wishes to hide his incision. Perhaps Ruben's draftsmanship is at fault or is that some kind of heresy! Indeed, there are other opinions on this, and here again the "diagnosis" can be said to depend on the eye of the beholder. A group of Spanish authors see evidence of cancer in the left breast of the figure on the right. [2] They cite retraction of the left nipple, smaller total volume of the left breast than the right, irregular tumour with skin redness suggesting inflammatory disease and visible nodes in the left axilla. Why not make your own "diagnosis" if your travels ever take you to the Prado museum in Madrid where the painting is housed?

References

[1] Rembrandt's eyes, Simon Schama, Alan Lane the Penguin Group, London 1999.

[2] GrauJ., Estape J., Diaz-Padron M. Breast cancer in Rubens paintings. *Breast cancer Research and Treatment*, 68, 89-93, 2001.

Theodora

Theodora, the wife of the great Roman Emperor Justinian (527-565 CE), one of the most cultured and learned emperors of his era, was famous in her own right. She seems to be an "icon" in more ways than one, literally in terms of the style of the mosaic from the Basilica San Vitale, Ravenna, and figuratively, for what she represents for women with power (the political power she shared with her husband Justinian). According to several accounts, she died from breast cancer, although this is debated. [1] She also is said to have refused mastectomy, understandable perhaps given the lack of anaesthesia at the time, but also seen by some as refusing disfigurement.

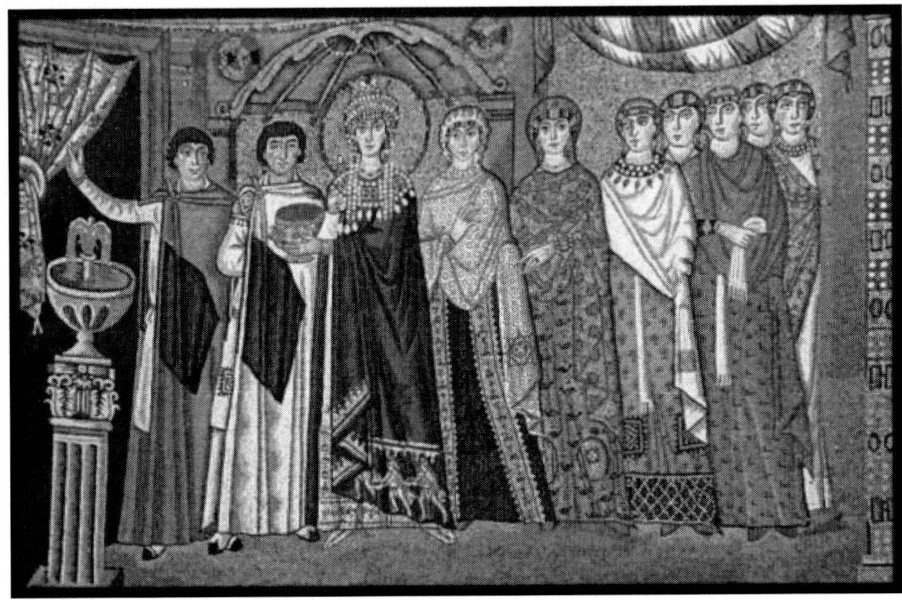

Empress Theodora, Mosaic in Basilica San Vitale.

It is well known that Theodora's life was immoral before her marriage and she had indeed performed in the theatre of the hippodrome and then worked in the brothels of the east, especially in Alexandria.

Furthermore, it is known that, when she was going to marry the Imperial heir Justinian (523 CE), the Emperor Justin I abolished the law that prohibited marriage between members of the senatorial class and prostitutes. On the other hand, it is also clear that the life of Theodora was morally irreproachable after her marriage. Procopius, [2] describing the Empress' appearance during her last years, wrote that her earlier beautiful and cheerful face showed paleness; furthermore, an expression of fatigue and melancholy was apparent in her contemporary portrayals, such as in the famous mosaic already mentioned. The African Bishop Victor Tonnennensis, contemporary of the Empress, confirms in his ``Chronicle" [3] that Theodora died of breast cancer which had metastasized all through her body: ``*Theodora Augusta Calchedonensis Synodi inimica canceris plaga corpore toto perfusa vitam prodigiose nivit."*

The Byzantine physicians Aetius [4] (sixth century) knew well the existence of breast cancer and considered it to be the most common form of cancer amongst middle-aged women. He also described the techniques of total mastectomy. The suggestion from historical sources indicates that Theodora's cancer was inoperable the nature of which her contemporary, Aetius, sets out clearly in his text, "tight attachment of the tumor to the thorax; thus making removal of the diseased breast from the healthy area a dangerous operation". [4] My personal view would be that whether or not she submitted herself to surgery her treatment would have been dictated to the teachings of Galen. Galen, (2ndC AD) who studied in Alexandria and practiced in Rome, became the most influential physician of the then known world. He extended the Hippocratic humoural theory of disease and taught that cancer was related to the accumulation of an excess of black bile (melancholia) that coagulated in the breast. He supported this view by suggesting that women clear themselves of black bile during their monthly periods and therefore after the menopause they are no longer cleansed. This conveniently explained the increasing incidence of breast cancer amongst women in their fifth and sixth decades. If such was the case it would appear logical to cleanse the women again by repeated purgation and bleeding, coupled with diets with a low capacity of producing black bile. It is a piece of almost black comedy to read how those ancient surgeons hazarding amputation of the breast were encouraged not to stop the bleeding too quickly in order to allow the excess of evil humours to escape.

Acknowledgments

I am much in debt to the scholarly researches of John Lascaratos and Effie Poulakou-Rebelakou, from the Department of the History of Medicine, University of Athens, for providing direction for my research on the Ravenna mosaic.

References

[1] Browning R. Justinian and Theodora. London: Thames and Hudson, 1987: 165±178. 1999 Blackwell Science Ltd.

[2] Mantellou P. The personal life of Theodora before her marriage with Justinian, according to Procopius' Anecdota. *Byzantine Studies* 1990; 2: 330±339.

[3] Mommsen T, ed. Victoris Tonnennensis episcopi Chronica. In: Monumenta Germaniae Historica, Vol. II. Berolini: Weidmann, 1894: 202.
[4] Zervos S, ed. Aetii Sermo Sextidecimus et Ultimus. Leipzig: A Mangkos, 1901: 60±68.

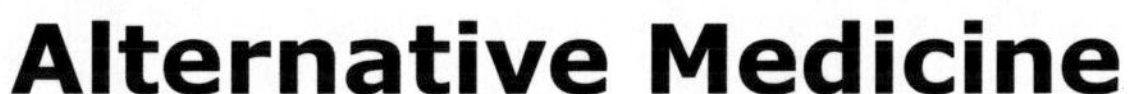

Alternative Medicine

Chapter 12

An Open Letter to HRH the Prince of Wales: With Respect Your Highness You've Got It Wrong

(BMJ 2004; 329:118)

Your Royal Highness,

20 years ago, on the occasion of the 150th anniversary of the British Medical Association (BMA), you were appointed our President and used your position to admonish my profession for its complacency. You also took advantage of this platform to promote "alternative" medicine. Shortly after that I enjoyed the privilege of meeting with you at a series of colloquia organized by the Royal Society of Medicine (RSM) to debate the role of complementary and alternative medicine (CAM) in health care.

Of course you won't remember me but the event is indelible in my memory. I was the only one amongst my professional colleagues to unequivocally register dissent. At the cocktail party to mark the closure of our meetings I had the impertinence to say that although I disagreed with you about "alternative" medicine you were absolutely right about the architects. (I'm sure you remember the "carbuncle" episode). Quick as a flash you described how the previous night, having dinner at the Royal Institute of

British Architects (RIBA), you were accosted by a prominent architect who stated that you were absolutely wrong about British architecture but he couldn't agree more about your stand on British Medicine! From that point onwards you won my undying devotion.

A few days later you were rewarded with a four-page supplement in the London Evening Standard, promoting unproven cures for cancer and I was invited by the same journal to respond. I requested the same space but was only allowed one page, which at the last minute was cut by a quarter to make space for an advert for a new release by "Frankie Goes to Hollywood". Furthermore the sub-editors embarrassed me with banner headline, "With respect your Highness, you've got it wrong". (The Standard August 13th 1984). As I have nothing more to lose I'm happy for that headline to grace the BMJ today.

Over the last 20 years I have treated thousands of patients with cancer and lost some dear friends and relatives along the way with this dreaded disease. I guess that for the majority of my patients their first meeting with me was as momentous and memorable as mine was with you. Sadly, however hard I try, many of these courageous men and women are not instantly recognized and covertly I check their notes before each follow up in order to practice the benign deception of greeting them like long lost friends. This phenomenon of asymmetrical relationships I like to describe as the "gradient of power". The power of my authority comes with a knowledge built on 40 years of study and 25 years of active involvement in cancer research. I'm sensitive to the danger of abusing this power and as a last resort I know that the General Medical Council (GMC) is watching over my shoulder to ensure I respect a code of conduct with a duty of care that respects patient's dignity and privacy and reminds me that my personal beliefs should not prejudice my advice.

If you will forgive me Sir, your power and authority rests on an accident of birth. Furthermore as illustrated above, your public utterances are worthy of four pages, whereas if lucky I might warrant one. I don't begrudge you that authority and we probably share many opinions about Art and Architecture, but I do beg of you to exercise your power with extreme caution when advising patients with life threatening diseases to embrace unproven therapies. There is no equivalent of the GMC for the monarchy, so it is left to either sensational journalists or more rarely the quiet voice of loyal subject such as myself, to warn you that you may have overstepped the mark. It is in the nature of your world to be surrounded by sycophants (including members of the medical establishment hungry for their mention in the Queen's birthday honours list) who constantly reinforce what they assume are your prejudices.

Sir, they patronize you! Allow me this chastisement. Last week I had a sense of *déjà-vu*, when you welcomed the BMA representatives to Llandudno for the annual meeting and later appeared in The Observer (June 27th) and Daily Express (June 28th) promoting coffee enemas and carrot juice for cancer.

Much has changed since you shocked us out of our complacency 20- years ago. The GMC is reformed and, as part of this revolution, so has our undergraduate teaching. Professional development is part of our student's core curriculum, involving modules in the Humanities. Students are taught the importance of the spiritual domain but at the same time study the epistemology of Medicine, or in simpler words the nature of proof. Many lay people have an impressionistic notion of science as a cloak for bigotry. Nothing could be further from the truth. The scientific method is based on the deductive process that starts with the humble assumption that your hypothesis might be wrong and is then subjected to experiments that carry the risk of falsification. This approach works. For example in my own specialist disease, breast cancer, we have witnessed a 30% fall in mortality since 1984, resulting from a worldwide collaboration in clinical trials, accompanied by improvements in quality of life as measured by psychometric instruments. You promote the Gerson diet whose only support comes from inductive logic i.e. anecdote. I have Gerson's book on my desk as I write.

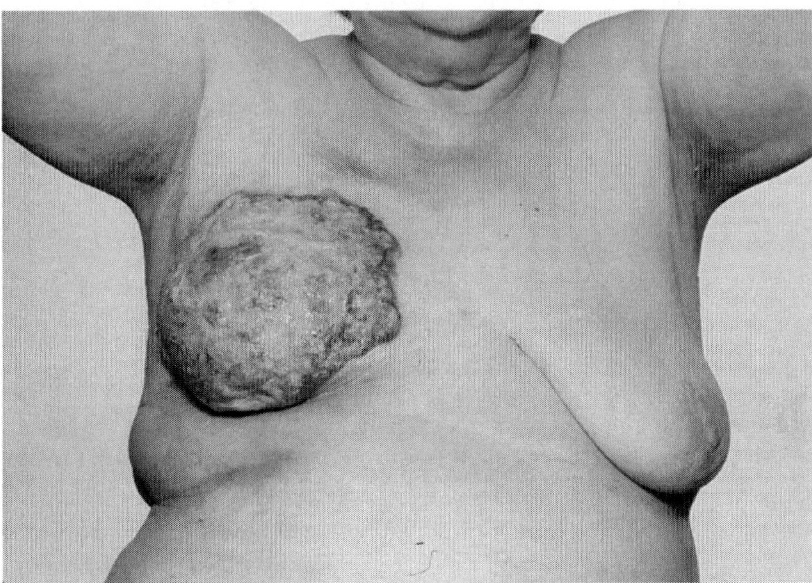

Locally advanced breast cancer.

Forget the implausible rationale; simply search for anything other than testimonial support. What is wrong with anecdote you may ask? After all these are real human-interest stories. The problems are manifold but start with the assumption that cancer has a predictable natural history. "The patient was only given 6 months to live, tried the diet and lived for years". This is an urban myth. None of us are so arrogant as to predict that which is known only to the Almighty. With advanced breast cancer the ***median*** expectation of life might be 18 months, but many of my patients live for many years longer, with or without treatment. I have always advocated the scientific evaluation of CAM using controlled trials and if "alternative" therapies pass these rigorous tests of so called "orthodox" medicine, then they will cease to be alternative and join our armamentarium. If their proponents lack the courage of their convictions to have their pet remedies subjected to the "hazards of refutation" then they are the bigots who will forever be condemned to practice on the fringe.

I have much time for *complementary* therapy that offers improvements in quality of life or spiritual solace, providing that it is truly integrated with modern medicine, but I have no time at all for "alternative" therapy which places itself above the laws of evidence, and practices in a metaphysical domain that harks back to the dark days of Galen. The "post-modern" philosophers, with their talk of post-Enlightenment hegemony, would have us believe that all knowledge is relative and the dominance of one belief system is determined by the power of its proponents. The hazards of this way of thinking are beautifully exposed in Francis Wheen's new book, "How Mumbo-Jumbo conquered the World". Instead, perhaps we should all remain cognizant of the words of the Nobel Lauriat, Jaques Monod; "Personal self-satisfaction is the death of the scientist. Collective self-satisfaction is the death of the research. It is restlessness, anxiety, dissatisfaction, agony of mind that nourish science". Please your Royal Highness; help us nourish medical science by sharing our agony.

Yours Sincerely,

Michael Baum

Chapter 13

Book Review "Whole Person Care: A New Paradigm for the 21st Century"

Tom A. Hutchinson
Editor

(Focus on Alternative and Complementary Therapies
Volume 17, Issue 2, pages e17–e19, June 2012)

This will be an unusual book review because it says just as much about the reviewer as the reviewed. Let me tell you a little 'about myself and the relevance of this to the book review that will become apparent if you stay with me for a paragraph or two.

I was a little boy at the time of the London Blitz and to escape the bombs my family translocated to Birmingham. I went to the local grammar school and studied medicine at the local medical school. I was always ambitious to become a surgeon and completed my surgical training at Kings College Hospital in London. I was fortunate to be appointed professor of surgery there in 1980 and since then have served as professor of surgery at the Royal Marsden Hospital and University College London. After retiring from my clinical chair I was appointed visiting professor in medical humanities.

Halfway through my career as a general surgeon I opted to specialize in the management and research of carcinoma of the breast. It always irritates me when critics suggest that a specialist becomes very narrow in his focus and that although I would know an awful lot about the breast and its cancer, I would know little of the patient as a whole. Nothing could be further from the truth; my specialization in fact broadened my interest and widened my perspective.

As a clinical scientist I became interested in the philosophy of science and from this developed my lasting interest in clinical trials. I started off as a dilettante in this field but ultimately was treated seriously and was rewarded with the accolade of delivering the Karl Popper Memorial lecture at the London School of economics. [1]

My clinical practice taught me the importance of communication skills and forced me to confront the ethical dilemma of entering patients with breast cancer into clinical trials. The empathy I developed from confronting the fears and suffering of women with breast cancer persuaded me to recruit clinical psychologists. My team, together with Prof Lesley Fallowfield, helped establish the sub discipline of psychosocial oncology. I was rewarded for these efforts by being appointed as the first chairman of the psychosocial oncology committee of our National Cancer Research Institute. Out of this area of interest I became aware of how many of my patients were turning to alternative medicine as a modality for supporting them through the trials and tribulations of the diagnosis and management of breast cancer. I therefore studied the social anthropology of complementary and alternative medicine. In recognition of my efforts in this field I was asked to chair a committee on behalf of the European Society of Mastology (EUSOMA) looking into the role of complementary and alternative medicine in patients with breast cancer. [2] We concluded that there was only one kind of medicine; that which worked. "Alternative medicine", as far as I was concerned was simply medicine that did not work. However, I realized that there were unmet needs of patients with cancer that had to be addressed. The answer to this problem was not bogus quackery but good medicine that included empathy, good communication skills and psychological and spiritual support. Furthermore, I became dismayed at the way the English language was hijacked by the proponents of quack remedies to disguise what was on offer. I resented the word "healing" because it was a weasel word that disguised the fact that alternative medicine failed to change the natural course of life threatening diseases, I also resented the way that "holistic medicine" was introduced as another concept to disguise the fraud of what was on offer by proponents of alternative medicine. In fact the very use of the word holistic, demonstrated that these people simply did not understand the meaning of holon/holistic and confused it with "whole". I even delivered an eponymous lecture on "Concepts of holism in Orthodox and alternative medicine", at the Royal College of physicians in London.[3]

Ultimately my heavy workload, and the fact that I was dealing with cancer, lead to a period of acute depressive illness. I was indeed "the wounded healer".

That's enough about me now let's look at the book. From the start the title and subtitle of the book, "Whole person care: A new paradigm for the 21st century", had me screaming silently in my study and throwing the book across the room. My initial reaction was; "Here we go again, trying to teach me what whole person care was about without understanding the difference between "holistic" and "whole" and then having the temerity to abuse the concept of the paradigm shift to claim that this was something new". I was about to refuse the invitation to review of the book but before doing so I thought, at least I should read the forward. My pre-judgment of this book was totally wrong and I apologize. In my defense I think it is a most unfortunate choice of title and subtitle, but I quickly learnt where the editor, Tom Hutchinson, was coming from. Tom Hutchinson truly does understand his scientific philosophy and is using the word paradigm in its correct context according to the teachings of Thomas Kuhn. Furthermore, when he is using "whole" he does indeed mean ***whole*** and not confusing it with holon/holistic. In the first chapter he defines what the whole person and whole person care mean. "Whole person care is not knowing all about the patient in all dimensions, biological, physiological, social and spiritual. Such an undertaking is doomed to failure …when the patient comes to see a doctor he does not expect a combination biological scientist, psychologist, social worker and spiritual guidance counselor… within the context of the clinical interaction he or she wants someone who will provide competent medical care and treat him seriously as a person usually no more and no less." He then goes on to define the word healing, central to these discussions in this book, in a manner that I find acceptable and again I would like to quote. "Curing versus healing are not just different, they are diametrically opposed. For instance the goal of the patient in the curing mode is survival. This is not limited to physical survival but also extends to survival of all that the patient has learned to identify as himself including physical appearance and lifestyle relationships and everything else that makes up a life, in other words the goal is to avoid change. Healing comes from the acceptance of change. This acceptance allows the patient to grow to a new sense of himself as a person, perhaps with the disease, with a new experience of integrity and wholeness that is different to the old status quo." In other words in the healing mode the power shifts away from the doctor to the patient, furthermore the physician's role in the healing has to depend on his particular gifts and characteristics as a person and on the particular gifts and characteristics of the patient. It was for this reason that I spent the first half of my review talking about myself. Everyone who is a clinical practitioner reading this book, to do it justice, has to approach the subject with self-awareness and self-criticism.

It is important to appreciate that this book is really a philosophy of the doctor/patient relationship and not a textbook of medicine. There is an excellent chapter by Eric Cassell, describing the concept of suffering in a rather beautiful philosophical manner that appealed to me. Again I would like to quote: "Suffering has most commonly been associated with pain or other physical symptoms. It is now generally accepted however that pain or other symptoms and suffering, are distinct. People with no symptoms may suffer. Suffering is the specific distress that occurs when persons feel their intactness or integrity as persons threatened or disintegrating, and it continues until the threat is gone or impact on us or intactness is restored".

There is another chapter that is entitled, "The healing journey", which is also a rather neat philosophical debate on the nature of personhood and the nature of healing. It starts off with the fact that the "human condition" and the meaning of life are difficult concepts for the individual patient to live with even when they are well and each will react in a unique way when they are sick. This then provides the doctor a unique platform or canvas upon which to work at the time of disease or suffering of the person in question. "Perhaps the real goal of medicine should be to support patients on their healing journey, to help patients move towards a life with greater sense of connection and meaning and a new relationship to wounding and suffering." I considered at this point that the author was beginning to suggest that the doctor takes on the role of the priest or shaman in a secular society. I have no objection to this providing the clinician is trained to do so and perhaps the importance of this book is that it does indeed provide the training for a new role of the doctor in the doctor-patient relationship. I also began to speculate whether this kind of whole person care might provide precisely what the proponents of alternative medicine are offering but without the humbug and false promises. In fact I would go further and suggest that if all our young undergraduates and postgraduates were taught the philosophy embedded in this book, we would begin to see the end of the alternative medicine industry.

Along the way there are a number of passages in the book that describe the "wounded healer" and I recognize myself in these passages. I accept the criticism that we have an ethical obligation to our patients for self-care, which is not a luxury but a clinical imperative. In that black period of my life where I suffered from acute depression I was not providing a good clinical service neither could I fulfill the role as *pater familiaris*.

Inevitably there was the chapter on complementary and alternative therapies and inevitably this section provided anecdotal evidence as to how insensitive and awful doctors are and how much better we would be if we offered quack remedies. This wasn't stated explicitly but, as frequently seen these days, the provision of quack cures is disguised as "integrative medicine". Integrative medicine, as far as I'm concerned, is a way of sneaking in alternative medicine whilst at the same time practicing real medicine. It's a pity that this apologia for alternative medicine was allowed into a book, which is otherwise a rather beautiful and sensitive philosophical discussion on the nature of personhood, suffering and healing.

12 months ago my wife underwent major surgery to decompress her cervical spine, without which she would have ended up in a wheelchair. I will be forever indebted to the technical skills of the surgeon involved, but it was left to me, perhaps appropriately, to care for her during the period of healing and rehabilitation.

The stress of all this precipitated episodes of acute angina and I then underwent an urgent angioplasty with two stents placed into my coronary arteries. I was once again indebted to the technical skills of my doctor and the research and development beforehand that allowed my coronary arteries to be dilated and held open via a small incision in my right wrist. Whilst I was recovering my cardiologist came in for a chat and I asked him when I could return to my normal life. He replied, "You never had a *normal life* Mike and I need to persuade you to recognize that your attitudes and work ethic, has driven you to this point. Please re-evaluate your goals and define what is truly important in your life." I have spent the last 12 months following this advice, I feel completely rehabilitated and whole again, my only disappointment was that this process should have started 20 years earlier.

In conclusion, this is very interesting and worthwhile book which is essentially a treatise on the philosophy of the doctor-patient relationship and it should find its place in the training of young doctors and in the fullness of time, if the lessons contained within this book were assimilated, then I would predict that *alternative* medicine would wither on the vine.

References

[1] http://www2.lse.ac.uk/publicEvents/pdf/20071106_Popper.pdf

[2] Baum M, Cassileth BR, Daniel R, Ernst E, Filshie J, Nagel GA, Horneber M, Kohn M, Lejeune S, Maher J, Terje R, Smith WB. The role of complementary and alternative medicine in the management of early breast cancer: recommendations of the European Society of Mastology (EUSOMA). *Eur J Cancer*. 2006 Aug;42(12):1711-4.

[3] Baum M, Concepts of holism in orthodox and alternative medicine. *Clinical Medicine* 2010, 10; 37-40.

Chapter 14

Concepts of Holism in Orthodox and Alternative Medicine

The Samuel Gee Lecture

Royal College of Physicians

April 6th 2009

(Published in Clinical Medicine 2010, Vol 10, No 1: 37–40)

Abstract

In this essay I explore the nature of holism in orthodox and alternative medicine and illustrate the true meaning of the words with a complicated case history concerning the life or death of a young pregnant mother suffering from a BRCA type breast cancer. I conclude Holism in medicine is an open ended and exquisitely complex understanding of human biology that over time has lead to spectacular improvements in the length and quality of life of patients with cancer and that this approach encourages us to consider the transcendental as much as the cell and molecular biology of the human organism. "Alternative" versions of holism are arid and closed belief systems, locked in a time warp, incapable of making progress yet quick to deny progress in the field of scientific medicine.

Introduction

It is always a particular honour to be invited to deliver an eponymous lecture.

Samuel Gee in whose memory I have been asked to deliver this paper, shared two things in common with me. First he worked at University College London and so did I, secondly he was personal physician to the Prince of Wales a role I might have enjoyed had I not been so outspoken about holistic medicine. (1)

The art and science of the practice of medicine have the twin objectives of improving length of life and quality of life. (2) All other outcome measures must be considered surrogates and discounted from this discussion. The objective of this paper is to illustrate how the clinician himself can be an holistic practitioner contributing much to the quality of life, even amongst those patients who are pre-determined to die but also to recognise the limits of his skills and to know when to call upon other agents skilful in the practice of complementary care.

Holism As a Word and a Concept

General Jan Smuts coined the word 'holism' in 1926, using the word to describe the tendency in nature to produce wholes from the ordered grouping of units. The philosopher and author Arthur Koestler developed the idea more fully in his seminal book 'Janus: A Summing-Up', (3) in which he talks about self-regulating open hierarchic order (SOHO). 'Biological holons are self-regulating open systems which display both the autonomous properties of wholes and the dependent properties of parts. This dichotomy is present on every level of every type of hierarchical organisation and is referred to as the Janus Phenomenon.'

Holism in the Organisation of Organic Systems

To do justice to Jan Smuts' definition of the word holism, we have to start with a "reductionist" approach to the molecular level, and then from these basic building blocks attempt to reconstruct the complex organism which is the human subject living in harmony within the complex structure of a modern democratic Nation state. Since Watson and Crick described the structure and function of DNA in 1953, the development of biological holism has grown way beyond anything Jan Smuts might have envisaged. The basic building block of life has to be a sequence of DNA that codes for a specific protein. These DNA sequences or genes are organised within chromosomes forming the human genome. The chromosomes are packed within the nucleus with an awe-inspiring degree of miniaturisation. The nucleus is a holon looking inwards at the genome and outwards at the cytoplasm of the cell. The cell is a holon that looks inwards at the proteins which guarantee its structure and function contained within its plasma membrane, and at the energy transduction pathways contained within the mitochondria which produce the fuel for life. As a holon, the cell looks outwards at neighbouring cells of a self-similar type which may group together as glandular elements, but the cellular holon also enjoys cross-talk with cells of a different developmental origin communicating by touch through tight junctions, or by the exchange of chemical messages via short-lived paracrine polypeptides. These glandular elements and stromal elements group together as a functioning organ which is holistic in looking inwards at the exquisite functional integrity of itself, and outwards to act in concert with the other organs of the body. This concert is orchestrated at the next level in the holistic hierarchy through the neuro-endocrine/immunological control mediated via the hypothalamic pituitary axis, the thyroid gland, the adrenal gland, the endocrine glands of sexual identity, and the lympho-reticular system that can distinguish self from non-self. Even this notion of self is primitive compared with the next level up the hierarchy where the person exists in a conscious state somewhere within the cerebral cortex, with the mind, the great unexplored frontier, which will be the scientific challenge of doctors in the new millennium.

The Modern Oncologist As a Holistic Practitioner

A modern oncologist is one member of a team. Any self-respecting team these days includes a surgical oncologist, clinical oncologist, medical oncologist, diagnostic radiologist, histopathologist and clinical nurse specialist/counsellor. It is my particular prejudice that the clinical nurse specialist (nurse counsellor) bridges the gap between the clinical scientist and those other disciplines that offer complementary and supportive care. My own team has immediate access to a clinical psychologist, as well as counsellors and I have made attempts in the past to evaluate this service according to scientific principles, with the development and use of psychometric tools. (4).

I therefore wish to illustrate these abstract concepts with a clinical case history that demanded all the powers and expertise of a multidisciplinary team to come up with an appropriate management plan.

The Story of Mrs Sarah G aged 29 Years

- This young woman was asymptomatic but presented to my clinic following the detection of a suspicious abnormality on mammographic screening. Fine needle aspiration cytology confirmed the diagnosis of breast cancer.
- There was no relevant past medical history and she was gravid 1 para 1
- There was a significant family medical history. She was of Ashkenazi Jewish origin. Her mother died of breast cancer at the age of 36 and her sister was recently diagnosed with bilateral breast cancer at the age of 21. A paternal aunt had breast cancer at the age of 37.
- On clinical examination she was a fit young woman and the only abnormality of note was an area of ill-defined nodularity in the upper outer quadrant of her right breast.
- Special investigations were reviewed. The mammograms, which she had for screening, because of her family history, showed an area of microcalcifications in the upper outer quadrant of the right breast. Fine needle aspiration cytology showed atypical cells but a core cut biopsy showed duct carcinoma in-situ and also areas of invasive duct cancer of intermediate grade.
- In the interval between diagnosis and the planning of surgery, the patient mentioned that she had missed a period and pregnancy testing was positive.
- How should this patient be treated and what should we do about her pregnancy?

****

The simple stereotype way by which I have presented the case history was intentional. Nothing but the patient's true narrative of her own life experience and fears can do justice to this story. We must recognize that her mother died young and as a result an aunt raised her. We must also try to understand what it must feel like to be forced to come to terms with one's mortality at such an early age and the clinical history alone cannot do justice to the strength of feeling of Sarah and her husband about producing a sibling for their little daughter, in other words the pregnancy is very precious.

Next we come to the major ethical issues that are raised by this case. From her family tree and Ashkenazi origins it is highly likely that there is a germ line mutation in the BRCA1 or BRCA2 gene. Sarah had already been counselled on this matter, hence her exposure to mammographic screening, yet she had opted not to go forward for the genetic test because at the time there was no proven intervention, if she had tested positive. Now her own cancer has made it even more likely that this extended family has a germ line mutation, putting increasing pressure on other female relatives for genetic testing. This leads on to a further consideration of the genotype of the foetus. Would she want to know if it was male or female and abort the female? Might it be possible to test for the gene on a cell of the developing foetus if a female and abort the female foetus if the test is positive? What about IVF and embryo selection? Unfortunately our ethical guidelines on these difficult issues are falling far behind the rapid pace of progress at the molecular level. (5)

Next the issue of abortion itself: is this ethical or unethical? Well this of course depends very much on the cultural and religious background of her family. In a largely secular Society most patients would consider themselves rational humanists and therefore feel that they should be fully autonomous in this decision. Yet if the patient were Catholic then abortion would be considered a sin whereas, according to the Jewish faith if the abortion would prolong her life by even a day then it might be considered an ethical imperative to proceed with the abortion. This immediately brings us back to the issue of epistemology. Although in theory it is plausible that the continuation of the pregnancy may increase the rate of progression of her breast cancer, are there empirical data that support or refute that opinion? In fact, the weight of evidence would suggest that if anything women with breast cancer who become pregnant have a better outcome than expected, once again illustrating the beauty of the deductive logic whereby a plausible hypothesis is overturned by the accumulation of empirical data. Whilst on the subject of epistemology we then have to consider the evidence for and against different treatment modalities in this case and also be in a position to weigh up the balance between quality of life and length of life, as a result of these different treatments. It so happens we have an enormous weight of evidence that will help Sarah with her decision making process about treatment. We know with confidence that conservative surgery supplemented by radiotherapy will provide the same chance of cure as more radical surgery. We now know that adjuvant systemic chemotherapy in young women with breast cancer significantly prolongs life. But what about the effect of chemotherapy on the foetus? Again it is plausible that chemotherapy may have such an adverse effect on the foetus that in order to provide the patient with the best chance of survival the foetus should be aborted, yet empirical data suggest that once organogenesis is complete, the foetus is remarkably robust and can in fact tolerate chemotherapy. So if the continuation of her pregnancy is not likely to interfere with treatment and thus impair her length of life and if the foetus is tolerant of the treatment, then the only matter left to consider for this precious pregnancy is the possibility of Sarah dying young, leaving a second orphaned child to be brought up by Sarah's husband. However painful it was for me as a personal physician, I felt that it was my responsibility to inform Sarah and her husband that breast cancer at the age of 29 has a very poor prognosis and whilst supporting their wish to continue with the pregnancy they needed to be aware of the dreadful possibility that the baby would be left without a mother. But then, as Sarah reminded me, she also grew up without a mother and her life to date has been fulfilled, whilst her husband's response demonstrated a nobility of spirit. He was prepared to shoulder the burden with the compensation that there would always be two sets of eyes to remind him of his beautiful wife. Finally, facing an uncertain future and coming to terms with her own mortality, Sarah needed spiritual and psychological support which was certainly beyond my own competence or even that of my nurse counsellor. In addition to her extended family and her Jewish faith we were able to call upon the agency of Chai-Lifeline, a volunteer organization set up specifically to work alongside doctors in this difficult and sensitive area.

Two years ago I attended the 5th birthday party of one of my grandchildren. In the midst of the mêlée I spotted Sarah with her cute little ginger haired green-eyed 5-year-old daughter. We exchanged meaningful glances, the only two in the room to fully understand the joy of this moment. Mother, daughter and surgeon were doing pretty well thank you.

To manage this case adequately required a working knowledge at all strata in the hierarchy that provides an holistic model of the human subject: understanding the failure of DNA repair mechanisms in BRCA I mutations at the molecular level, all the way up to the understanding of a woman in her central role as mother, wife and member of a faith community.

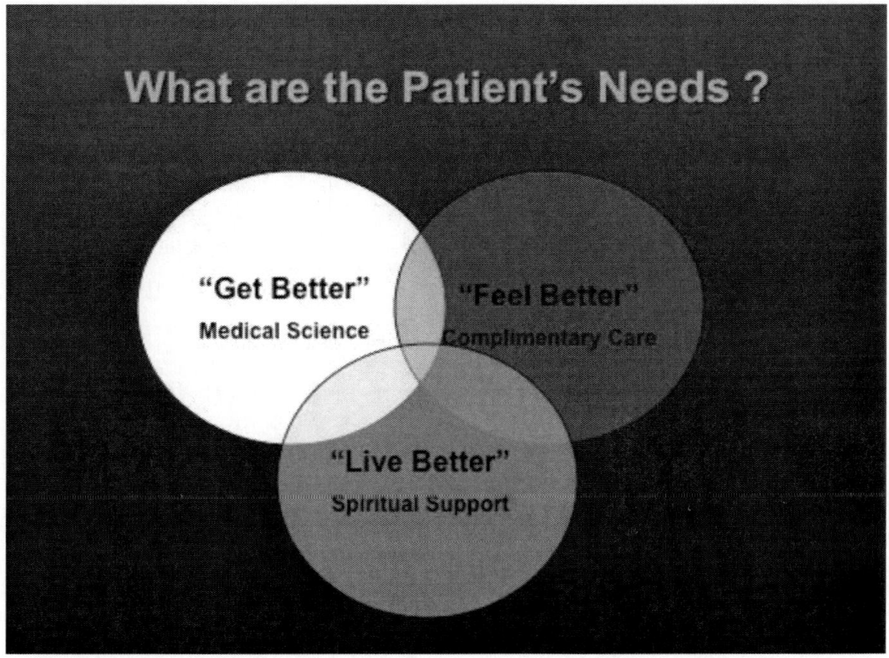

A simple model of a concept of holism that is relevant to a modern physician.

Conclusion

Holism in medicine is an open ended and exquisitely complex understanding of human biology that over time has led to spectacular improvements in the length and quality of life of patients with cancer. This approach encourages us to consider the transcendental as much as the cell and molecular biology of the human organism. Alternative versions of "holistic medicine" that offer claims of miracle cures for cancer by impossible dietary regimens, homeopathy or metaphysical manipulation of non existent energy fields, are cruel and fraudulent acts that deserve to be criminalized. Such "alternative" versions of holism are arid and closed belief systems, locked in a time warp, incapable of making progress yet quick to deny progress in the field of scientific medicine.

References

[1] Baum M, An Open Letter to HRH The Prince of Wales: With respect your Highness you've got it wrong. *BMJ* 2004; 329: 118.

[2] Calman, K and Downie, R. Why arts courses for medical curricula? *Lancet*, 1996; 347 : 1499 – 1500.

[3] Koestler, A. Janus: A summing up. Picador, London 1978.

[4] Fallowfield, L.J., Baum, M. Maguire G,P. Addressing the psychological needs of the conservatively treated breast cancer patient. *J.Roy.Soc.Med.* 80 (11): 646-700, 1987.

[5] Baum M, Pre-implantation genetic diagnosis (PGD): The spectre of eugenics or a ''no brainer'', *International Journal of Surgery* (2006) , 144145.

Chapter 15

Complementary and Alternative Medicine (CAM) within the National Health Service

(Paper delivered to the Royal College of General Practitioners 2006)

> "Doublethink means the power of holding two contradictory belief's in one's mind simultaneously, and accepting both of them"
>
> George Orwell, 1984

In his terrifying book 1984, George Orwell coined two terms that are useful starting points for this article, *doublethink* (see above) and *newspeak* which described a dilution and distortion of the English language sufficient to make the holding or communication of "subversive" thoughts impossible.

Newspeak is relevant to the semantics of this debate and *doublethink* relates to the nature of evidence and double standards that some would have us adopt.

Let us start with the semantics. CAM is nothing other than a shorthand device to start the discussion, shorthand for complementary and alternative medicine. To me "alternative" medicines are not only unproven (*vide infra)* but are also based on conceptual beliefs of human biology that are ancient, metaphysical and simply wrong. To think otherwise is to imply a denial of progress in our knowledge of human anatomy, physiology and biology.

Next we must consider the definition of "complementary". The Oxford English dictionary defines the word as, "that which completes or makes perfect, or that which when added completes a whole." In other words, whilst modern medical science struggles to cure patients, complementary medicine helps patients to feel better, and who knows, by feeling better the act of healing itself may be complemented. Some complementary approaches may be placebos, and the touch of the "healer" or the hand of the massage therapist could be guided by strange belief systems that are alien to modern science. Providing the intention is to support the clinician in his endeavours rather than compete in the relativistic market place of ideas one might set aside these concerns. Some of these complementary approaches might be in the psychosocial domain and others in the spiritual domain, acting as surrogates for religious faith in a secular society. [1] Even so, these interventions should be evidence based with outcome measures that reflect these important subjective and existential areas of experience. Examples of these might be psychological counselling, behaviour therapy, art therapy, music therapy, a favourable healing environment, therapeutic massage and even visits by the hospital chaplain. All of these have some evidence of efficacy and it is with some irony that I note that the psychometric instruments that quantify these subjective end-points were developed and are used in practice by orthodox medical practitioners ***not*** the proponents of alternative medicine. [2] It might also be worth mentioning that our National Cancer Research Institute has research development committees for complementary and psychosocial therapies. I chair the latter. I do not include homeopathy in this list as it has been debunked again and again [3,4,5] as nothing other than a placebo closer to witchcraft than science. [6] I have nothing intrinsically against placebo therapy that provides temporary relief but it's the intellectual dishonesty of homeopathy that I find so troubling.

This then brings us to the topic of *doublethink.* The department of health, the National Institute of Clinical Excellence (NICE), the Royal Colleges including the RCGP and the Medicines and Health products Regulatory Agency (MHRA) rightly demand evidence of efficacy and tolerability before endorsing treatments based on a very careful analysis of benefit, harm and cost. This is known as evidence based medicine (EBM).

EBM can be described as the systematic, explicit, conscientious and judicious use of the best available evidence when making healthcare decisions. In clinical medicine the most reliable evidence comes from controlled clinical trials that minimise bias. If such data are not available, EBM can also take into account other types of evidence. EBM is therefore applicable to all areas of medicine – including complementary medicine. EBM does not neglect individual experience, intuition, clinical judgement and patient preference. In clinical practice, evidence is merely one of several factors that go into a more complex equation for deciding which treatment is best for individual patients. Contrary to criticisms from the alternative lobby, EBM is not heartless or without compassion. To be guided by the best evidence means to give patients the best chances for getting better – what could be less "heartless" or more compassionate; ignorance based medicine (IBM)?

All human endeavours are prone to errors and, as research moves on, the evidence may change. Thus some treatments get better and some become obsolete. Like science, medicine deals with uncertainties, and the doctor has to choose the treatment with the least uncertainty given the prevailing circumstances for the patient. Also like science, EBM is always advancing and self-correcting. It is open to challenge by new discoveries. Pseudoscientific "medicine" largely stays the same.

As an illustration of this, homeopathy hasn't moved on for over 200 years, there are no "breakthroughs" in homeopathy and no homeopathic physician would be willing to design an experiment that might refute their precious belief system or accept the impartial judgement of others.

Or as J.R. Laidler pithily stated on his web page;

"You can never prove any alt-med claim false because you are biased, i.e. you don't already believe them. Only a person who is 'open-minded' can evaluate their claims in a fair and impartial manner. 'Open-minded' means 'willing to permanently suspend disbelief.' If you insist on holding on to your old, outmoded ideas, such as chemistry, biology, physics, anatomy, physiology or even simple logic, you will be blind to their new truth." [7]

This is what I would call "doublethink".

References

[1] Baum M, Ernst E, Lejeune S, Horneber M. The role of complementary and alternative medicine (CAM) in the care of patients with breast cancer. *European J Cancer* (in press 2006).

[2] Ebbs SR, Fallowfield LJ, Fraser SC, Baum M. Treatment outcomes and quality of life. *Int J Technol Assess Health Care*. 1989;5(3):391-400.

[3] Ernst E. A systematic review of systematic reviews of homeopathy. *Br J Clin Pharmacol* 2002;54:577-582.
[4] Shang A, Huwiler-Müntener K, Nartey L, et al. Are the clinical effects of homoeopathy placebo effects? Comparative study of placebo-controlled trials of homoeopathy and allopathy. *Lancet* 2005; 366: 726-732.
[5] The Lancet. The end of homoeopathy. *Lancet* 2005; 366: 690.
[6] Dominic Lawson Can you tell the difference between homeopaths and witch doctors? *The Independent*, Friday 26 May, 2006, 35.
[7] http://www.geocities.com/healthbase/altmed_debate_laidler.html?20065

Chapter 16

Can We Sustain an Open-Minded Approach to Homeopathy?

Commentary for the American Journal of Medicine 2009, 122, 973-974
Michael Baum and Edzard Ernst

The paper from the Office of Complementary and Alternative Medicine (OCCAM) of the NCI, has provoked us (open minded clinical scientists) to question the limits of an open mind. As chance would have it there was another Occam, William; a mediaeval monk considered to be the founding father of scientific philosophy. William of Occam's famous aphorism, known as Occam's razor, *"Essentia non sunt multiplicanda praeter neccessitatem"*, has come to mean that the simplest explanation that unifies multiple observations, "entities", is always the best. This is the principle of the diagnostic process where the best solution is the one that explains all the patient's symptoms, so that unlike homeopathy that treats multiple symptoms as separate entities, modern medicine treats the underlying pathology that creates all these symptoms. The second aphorism we like to quote is from our favourite American, Oliver Wendell Holmes, who stated in an essay lampooning homeopathy, (1) "Do you think I don't understand the hydrostatic paradox of controversy? If you had a bent tube, one arm of which was the size of a pipe-stem and the other big enough to hold the ocean, water would stand at the same height in one as in the other. Thus discussion equalizes fools and wise men in the same way, and the fools know it." In other words the evidence against homeopathy is the size of an ocean whilst the evidence in favour of homeopathy has the calibre of a pipe stem yet still we dignify it with an even handed debate. So is it a virtue to retain an open mind about homeopathy that starts from an absurd concept that dilutions of one molecule of a mother tincture in the volume of the solar system have therapeutic efficacy?

We understand the motive for OCCAM's office but feel justified to question the use of such scarce resources in such an unpromising area.

Coming to specifics of the paper published in this issue of Cancer. These cases were selected from 1260 managed by this clinic (1.1%). Yet the authors claim at the outset a 21% complete remission rate. In the end only 4 cases were considered worthy of report. Now 4 cases out of 14 would be interesting and would normally lead on to a formal phase II/III trial. However 4 cases out of 1260 (0.3%) is less interesting unless one believes in miracles. We have problems with miracles. Firstly, by definition they are very rare and it would therefore not be a good coping strategy for patients with advanced disease. Furthermore, miracles suggest divine intervention. What kind of divinity is it that judges who should benefit from the thousands of equally deserving cases?

Now we come to the crunch. We're as open minded as the next clinical scientist but our default position even with treatments based on rational physics, biology and physiology, has to be sceptical. These 4 cases are indeed "miracles" but as sceptics we have to look for rational explanations. First of all we are assured that the patients had no conventional therapy. Why should we believe that assertion? Patients rarely disclose that they are indulging in alternative therapy to orthodox practitioners; perhaps the reverse holds true as well.

Having said all that we still think it is appropriate and provocative for Cancer to have published this paper, not so much as to persuade people to believe in homeopathy but to question the spending of scarce resources on this type of work when OCCAM would be better off looking at herbal remedies where at least there is a half chance of an active ingredient being present at normal dilutions.

Personally we would go further and state that a belief in homeopathy exceeds the tolerance of an open mind. We think we must start from the premise that homeopathy cannot work and that any trials that are positive reflect publication bias or design flaws. Otherwise we must believe that water has a selective memory. So far homeopathy has failed to demonstrate efficacy in randomized clinical trials (RCT) and systematic reviews of well-designed studies [2,3]. Homeopathic physicians seem to clutch on to a series of poorly designed studies to retain their credibility or claim that the RCT is an inappropriate methodology to assess their belief system in the name of post modern relativism.[4,5] One might even question if any kind of evidence would persuade a homeopathic physician of the error of his ways.

Should we keep an open mind about astrology, perpetual motion, alchemy, alien abduction and sightings of Elvis Presley?

No, and we are happy to confess that our minds have closed down on homeopathy in the same way and here's why.

- Homeopathy is based on an absurd concept that denies progress in physics and chemistry. 160 years after "Homeopathy and Its Kindred Delusions", another essay by Oliver Wendell Holmes, we are still debating whether homeopathy is a placebo or not.[6]
- Homeopathy is only advocated for self-limiting conditions e.g. it cures a cold in seven days that would otherwise take a week. Do even homeopaths rely on their treatments for cancer and other life threatening conditions?
- There are no reported major "advances" in homeopathy.
- Homeopathic principles are "bold conjectures". There has been no spectacular corroboration of any of its founding principles. [7] An example of the spectacular corroboration of a bold conjecture is that the planet Pluto was predicted using Newtonian calculations and its discovery was counted as a spectacular corroboration of a bold conjecture. In medicine the same might apply to the discovery of antibiotics.

We are constantly reminded of Galileo's battle with the dogma of his day and how in the fullness of time this heretic was proven right.

The Galileo argument is a syllogism, a kind of logical argument in which one proposition (the conclusion) is inferred from two others (the premises) of a certain form. For example Van Gogh was a great artist not recognized in his lifetime. MB is an artist who has so far not sold a painting, ergo "He is great".

After more than 200 years we are still waiting for homeopathy "heretics" to be proven right whereas Galileo's genius was recognised not long after his death.

The true sceptic therefore takes pride in closed mindedness when presented with absurd assertions that contravene the laws of thermo-dynamics or deny progress in all branches of physics, chemistry, physiology and medicine.

As our old friend, the late lamented Petr Skrabanek, once stated, "if your mind is too open your brain slides out". Well our brains are too precious an organ to be hazarded in this way and our minds are tightly closed when asked to consider the possibility that homeopathy is anything other than placebos offered by a kindly practitioner with ample time at his disposal.

Reference

[1] Holmes, O. W. (1892) The Autocrat of the Breakfast Table ,40 Houghton Mifflin Boston.

Chapter 17

Homeopathy Waives the Rules-OK?

Spiked on Line 2006

Introduction

On September 1st 2006, The Medicines for Human Use (National rules for Homeopathic Products) Regulations Statutory Instrument 2006 No. 1952 came into force. As a headline that has an impact factor a little below “Small earthquake in Peru, few killed”. Yet by my reasoning this might be an early symptom of a malaise that is polluting our culture. The Medicines for Human Use Regulatory Agency (MHRA) came into being following the Medicines Act in 1968 to provide strict rules for licensing new medicines based on evidence of safety and efficacy following the thalidomide tragedy. All medicinal products on the market at that time were granted automatic product licences with the view of revisiting them in due course for evidence of safety and efficacy, but all new products had to pass these stringent rules. When Britain joined the common market in 1973, evidence of safety and efficacy for all medicines became mandatory except for homeopathy, which enjoyed a privileged place. However new homeopathic remedies could not be marketed, as they couldn’t provide efficacy data that would be required of conventional medicines. EC directive 2001/83 provided member states the opportunity to manage this discrepancy in the licensing of conventional and orthodox medicines. Sweden for example elected for a single standard of evidence, as a result of which new homeopathic remedies will never become available in that eminently rational country. By contrast, the UK Statutory instrument 2006 No. 1952 demonstrates that Britain no longer rules the waves but as far as homeopathy is concerned is prepared to waive the rules introducing a double standard of breathtaking *chutzpah.*[*]

As always the devil is in the detail and clouded in officialise.

Viz. Section 1 subsection 1(a)

- "An application for the grant of a UK marketing authorization for a national homeopathic product is not (my emphasis) required to be made in accordance with -(a) the second and third indents of Article 8.3(i) of the 2001 Directive, the requirement to submit results of pre-clinical and clinical trials".
- There again in Part 3 Evidence of efficacy, section 6 (c);
- "The data must consist of at least the results of investigations, commonly known as homeopathic "*provings*", which consist of the administration of a substance to a human subject in order to ascertain the symptoms produced by that substance."

Translated into English what that means is that homeopathy is spared from submitting the results of randomized controlled trials (RCTs) for evidence of efficacy but instead it would be acceptable to offer evidence obtained from "*provings*". Equal weight is therefore given to the evidence of scientific trials for modern medicines and *"Similia similibus curentur"* (the magic of similarities) for homeopathy.

Trial by Media

Friday September the 1st dawned with yet another morning of surrealistic debate over the airwaves followed by an afternoon and evening where art imitated life. I turned up at 07.00am in the studios of the Today programme with a sense of *déjà vu* all over again, to be cross examined by the presenter John Humphries and to be joined by the out of body voice of Dr. Fisher, spokesman for the Royal London Homeopathic Hospital (RLHH). There was nothing paranormal about his presence. It was just another example of the miracle of modern science whereby he could join us on air via electromagnetic waves transmitted from his cell phone in the wilds of Scotland, via some passing orbiting satellite to the studio and then out from there to the world at large. The most extraordinary comment from Dr. Fisher was an expression of satisfaction that at last homeopathy and orthodox medicine would be enjoying a level playing field! Eh?! I watched Arsenal draw with Middleborough one all, last Saturday at Highbury, in their beautiful new Emirates stadium. The playing field looked as level as a snooker table and at my count there were 11 men a side (although to be fair one of the 'Borough's defenders was sent off for the last 10 minutes of the game). How is it a level playing field for the Pharmaceutical Industry to have to submit the results of RCTs with thousands of patients, years of follow up, Good Clinical Practice (GCP) standards of governance and careful statistical analysis for efficacy and safety followed by a year or two of delay awaiting reports of cost-effectiveness from National Institute of Clinical Excellence (NICE), when all the homeopathy industry has to offer is the evidence that a substance, that is only retained in the "memory of water", can induce symptoms of a disease, if given in its natural state?

My next interview was on BBC breakfast television in the company of a charming young lady representing the society of homeopaths. She was brandishing a bottle of Arnica 30C, which she assured the viewing millions, was a proven remedy for bruising and minor trauma. Arnica is an extract of a yellow flower, *arnica Montana* and 30C means that it has been diluted in a volume larger than the Pacific Ocean. Although there is no plausible reason why it should work, my companion assured the audience that there was proof of its efficacy. Apart from the fact that all systematic reviews of RCTs have failed to show that any homeopathic remedy was anything other than a placebo [1,2,3,4,5], I happened to know of a trial of Arnica 30C carried out by the Blackie Foundation of the Royal London Homeopathic Hospital, for perineal trauma after traumatic births that gave negative results. I sat on their advisory board at the time and insisted that the trial should be published but it never was. When I challenged the young lady about this publication bias she was quick to boast that many negative trials for Arnica 30C had been published without realizing the contradiction she had just made.

Art Imitates Life

As chance would have it, I was meeting Professor Donald Marcus from Baylor University, for lunch that day, after which I took him to the National Gallery for a "ward round". He shares my interest in the teaching of medical humanities and I wanted to show him some of the paintings that I use to instruct medical students. Amongst the English 18C works we both admire is a delightful series by Hogarth, entitled "marriage a la mode". The last frame in this narrative shows the dying syphilitic wayward wife with her crippled syphilitic daughter clutching the hem of her dress. (Most of the characters in this morality play seem to be suffering from Sexually Transmitted Diseases). On one side of this picture we can witness the doctor and the apothecary indulging in a bout of fisticuffs. Hogarth completed this work in about 1742 when there was little to choose for lack of efficacy between the nostrums of the quacks and the potions of the doctor. Dr. Samuel Hahnemann "discovered" homeopathy about 50 years later and its initial success can be ascribed to the fact that the nothingness of homeopathy must have been preferable to the bleeding, cupping, leaches, purgation, laudanum and quicksilver provided by the university educated doctors of that period; In other words the placebo effect of the doctor's gravitas minus the toxic effects of his pharmacopoeia.

The following evening my wife and I attended a charity performance of Donizetti's "Lelisir d'amore". Donizetti was born in Northern Italy round about the time homeopathy was invented. In this comic opera (The Elixir of Love) an itinerant quack sells a potion that promises to make men irresistible to women. A local yokel is so convinced by its power that the placebo effect gives him the confidence to win back his long lost love. Donizetti sends up the placebo effects of quack remedies and the gullibility of a naïve public with delightful music and song. This work is as relevant now as it was when first performed. (Donizetti himself died a horrible, protracted death from syphilis, against which contemporary medicine was impotent.)

Does It Matter?

I have been accused by many of my good friends of wasting my time by "tilting at windmills" and will never win the argument. Maybe so-but I happen to believe that what we are witnessing is a very dangerous trend. I'm not out to win but only to fight the good fight. I think it both dangerous at a clinical level but even more so at a broader social level.

The Medical Dangers of Homeopathy

Most sceptics look upon homeopathy as a harmless placebo. Indeed that might be the case but the dangers of homeopathy are indirect. First, if a doctor knowingly perscribes a placebo, then he is guilty of deceit. There may be a case for such interventions for children but if used in adults it stinks of paternalism. Furthermore, when a kindly doctor offers evidence-based medicine the placebo effect comes with it unintentionally as an "add-on" for free.

Next, if homeopathy is licensed for the treatment of specific symptoms then that might encourage the patient to delay seeing the doctor and serious conditions might be overlooked.

Finally, the homeopathic remedies might be seen as an alternative to a proven treatment and individuals might be putting their life at risk. A recent example was seen in the BBC "Newsnight" production that showed that many pharmacies are marketing homeopathic anti-malarial preparations. This seems to have coincided with the experience of the London School of Hygiene and Tropical Medicine's experience with young back-packers coming back from Sub-Saharan Africa with acute malaria.

Sociological Dangers

I agree with my friendly critics, that even include my wife of 40 years, that I cannot win the argument. Neither do I think can the thousands of other like-minded rationalists bound together in the name of science. I can think of four explanations for my pessimism and they don't make edifying reading.

First there is the danger from within. I've noted an increasing tendency amongst young general practitioners to embrace the teachings of homeopathy. They have come to believe that this marks them out as modern, caring and open minded. How is it modern to embrace a belief system that is over 200 years old? Maybe in this topsy-turvy *Erewhon* world of ours it would be even more modern to embrace Galenic teachings again, as they are 1800 years old. (Incidentally the Gerson diet favoured as alternative therapy for cancer **is** neo-Galenism). How is it caring to offer placebos with deceitful intent? How is it open minded to accept a closed dogmatic belief that has conspicuously failed to describe any breakthroughs since its invention? The problem here is the medical profession itself is losing confidence in the scientific method and beginning to believe all the anti-science rhetoric of the tabloid media.

The next reason for my pessimism is the scientific illiteracy of the lay public that hasn't moved much since CP Snow spelt it out in his Rede Lecture (1959) "The two cultures and the Scientific Revolution".

"Closing the gap between our cultures is a necessity in the most abstract intellectual sense, as well as in the most practical. When those two senses have grown apart, then no society is going to be able to think with wisdom. For the sake of the intellectual life, for the sake of this country's special danger, for the sake of this Western society living precariously rich among the poor, for the sake of the poor who needn't be poor if there is intelligence in the world, it is obligatory for us to look at our education with fresh eyes."

Nearly 50 years later, if anything things have got worse. Fewer and fewer of our sixth formers are studying the sciences that they consider as too difficult and irrelevant. More and more are taking "soft options" such as sociology and media studies. Departments of Chemistry and Physics are now closing down in our Universities. Yet there is no expression of shame. Instead young people may take pride in their scientific illiteracy, blaming science for all the ills in the world and accusing science of spoiling this green and pleasant land. I'm not alone in thinking this, Lord Bragg, that great writer, broadcaster and polymath described these phenomena in his book "On Giants' Shoulders: Great Scientists and Their Discoveries from Archimedes to DNA", as did Lord Taverne in his book "The March of Unreason", and neither is a scientist.

This latter book also introduces my next concern and that is the growing power of post-modern relativism. The creeping success of this French school of philosophy with its impenetrable use of language has replaced the need for critical thought on our campuses.

As all systems of belief are equally valid, culturally determined and value laden then anything goes. It is now considered extremely bad form if I suggest I know more about breast cancer than a patient suffering from the disease. Furthermore, as it is a well known fact that there is a conspiracy of the Government, the Medical establishment and the Pharmaceutical industry to risk the health of young children with immunization regimens, then it is perfectly reasonable for the modern and caring "yummy mummy" to avoid this threat and protect their children with natural remedies. To argue otherwise is an expression of heuristic, triumphalistic, Western industrial bio-scientific global hegemony (or words to that effect).

My final concern relates to the opinion that belief in the irrational and supernatural are "hard wired" (genetically predetermined). This was a topic of debate at the British Association for Advancement of Science at the University of East Anglia in September this year. In a brilliant lecture, Professor Bruce Hood from the University of Bristol described an extraordinary series of experiments to demonstrate that scientists' efforts to combat "irrational" beliefs are ultimately futile. For example, even the most sceptical scientists would not swap their wedding rings for identical replicas. Attaching sentimental significance to inanimate objects is little different to belief in the supernatural. He argued that this capacity of the human mind to think intuitively and to develop theories had some evolutionary advantages: I disagree. Professor Lewis Wolpert of University College London wrote a beautiful little book as a primer for teaching scientific understanding, entitled "The Un-natural Nature of Science". That precisely is the point. Science is all about falsifying your theories, it is counter-intuitive and a completely un-natural way of viewing the world.

So what can be the evolutionary advantage for a belief in the supernatural?

I had been puzzling over this for sometime when a close friend of mine, Dr. Howard Herschon, a distinguished psychiatrist, provided the answer over a game of bridge. He argues this way: The bigger the tribe the more successful. With greater muscle the tribe can conquer neighbours, take more wives and cultivate more land. However this depends on having powerful leadership. A chieftain emerges who might be very clever or very strong in armed combat. He will reign supreme until he weakens or other alpha males start competing. This system then has inbuilt instability that might be described with chaos mathematical theory. Sooner or later the tribe will fragment into warring factions and be at risk of conquer by the neighbours. On the other hand, if their leader is a supernatural, omniscient and omnipotent being, then the tribe can only grow because no one can defeat their King.

In evolutionary terms one might expect *homo-scientificus*, who emerged at the Age of Enlightenment, to outpace and dominate *homo-sapiens*; after all, look at the fruits of scientific discovery; longer healthier lives, faster transport and instant world wide communication. Yet the scientific gene has built in the seeds of its own destruction. The fruits of science are available to all, the technological offspring of scientific discovery are available to all, which means the weapons of mass destruction (WMD) are available to all! If WMD get into the hands of un-evolved homo-sapiens and they wish to take over the world, in the name of their great and invisible chieftain, then G*D save us all!

Acknowledgments

I am indebted to Professor Raymond Tallis for his critique of an early draft of this manuscript and to Professor Edzard Ernst for teaching me about homeopathy.

References

[1] Linde K, Clausius N, Ramirez G, Melchart D, Eitel F, Hedges LV *et al.* Are the clinical effects of homoeopathy placebo effects? A meta-analysis of placebo-controlled trials. *Lancet* 1997;350:834-43.

[2] Ernst E. A systematic review of systematic reviews of homeopathy. *Br J Clin Pharmacol* 2002;54:577-82.

[3] Ernst E, Pittler MH, Stevinson C, White AR. The desktop guide to complementary and alternative medicine. Edinburgh: Mosby. 2001.

[4] Shang A, Huwiler-Muntener K, Nartey L, Juni P, Dorig S, Sterne JA *et al.* Are the clinical effects of homoeopathy placebo effects? Comparative study of placebo-controlled trials of homoeopathy and allopathy. *Lancet* 2005;366:726-32.

[5] Ernst E, Pittler MH, Wider B, Boddy K. The desktop guide to complementary and alternative medicine. 2nd edition. Edinburgh: Mosby/Elsevier. 2006.

Chapter 18

Magic Mushrooms and Bent Spoons: That Was the Week That Was!

(Healthwatch Newsletter July 2006)

The week beginning Monday the 22nd of May 2006 began cold and drizzly as if to warn me not to bother getting out of bed. The week ended with me thinking that the omens had been in part correct but had failed to include a surrealistic component in the auguries. On Monday every NHS health service trust responsible for commissioning both primary and secondary health care was sent a letter signed by me and 12 other scientist more distinguished than myself. These included seven Fellows of the Royal Society, one Nobel Laureate and the first Professor of complementary and alternative medicine (CAM) in the UK. In this letter we warned of the creeping acceptance of alternative medicine in the NHS, picking out homeopathy for special attention, otherwise known as "The Harry Potter School of Medicine". This is, of course, no joke as within the last couple of years the Royal London Homeopathic hospital was refurbished by the University College Hospitals Trusts (UCHT) after the expenditure of about £20,000,000.

As chance would have it, that very day, the National Institute of Clinical Excellence (NICE) gave conditional approval for the use of aromatase inhibitors (AIs) for postmenopausal women with hormone responsive tumours. I was particularly delighted by this news as I had personally lead much of the clinical research in this area over the last seven or eight years and reported the first positive results at a breast cancer conference in the USA in 2001. The Americans had adopted this treatment policy in 2003 but our NHS patients had to wait another three years. During this time the money spent on homeopathy in my own NHS trust, which happens to be UCHT, could easily covered the costs not only for the AIs but also *herceptin,* thus saving many lives through the practice of good evidence based medicine (EBM).

Someone then leaked our letter to the Times, and I awoke on Tuesday morning to a miasma of faecal material as *the shit hit the fan.* By some remarkable coincidence that day was also scheduled for his Royal Highness the Prince of Wales to address the assembly of the World Health Organization, on the merits of CAM.

My schedule that day looked something like this:

Miss breakfast
07.45 BBC Birmingham
08.00 BBC4 Today
08.30 BBC5
09.30 Start clinic with constant interruptions.
12.00 Operating theatre
Miss lunch
14.00 More patients
15.15 BBC world service
16.30 ITN news interviewed for 20 minutes outdoor in the rain
17.30 Sky news live
18.00 Pick up message from husband of patient of mine who has just been diagnosed with liver metastases.
19.00 Quick dinner
20.00 Meet said husband for a malt whiskey or three for consolation and shoulder to cry on. (It worked both ways)

On Wednesday the backlash began, with the correspondence columns and most of the op eds, falling over each other in describing our stand as that of heartless scientists, closed minded bigots and Jurassic doctors. On the last point I was amused to note that in the Prince's speech he urged the audience to respect ancient wisdom. Perhaps our aggregate wisdom of about 700 years wasn't ancient enough or perhaps our failing was that we were all of white European stock. It took a pretty thick skin not to be upset by the amazing scientific illiteracy of our critics.

On Thursday I was back in my clinic. My first patient was a lovely Chinese lady in her mid forties. She had come to see me a few weeks earlier for a second opinion. Three years ago she had been treated for breast cancer with breast conserving surgery, radiotherapy and tamoxifen. She had now recurred close to the original site. Her original surgeon wanted to carry out a mastectomy but I had been able to salvage her breast. This was her first post-operative visit. She was of course delighted that the operation had been a success but because of all the publicity she "confessed" rather sheepishly, to taking traditional Chinese medicine alongside tamoxifen for three years. She described it as magic mushrooms that boost the immune system and I have since learnt that they are indeed a mushroom extract known as Ganoderma sporo-pollen and ganoderma spore bioactive lipids. If anyone out there can let me know if this stuff can compete for the oestrogen receptor or interfere with the action of the enzymes that convert tamoxifen to 4-Hydroxy-N-Desmethyltamoxifen, the active metabolite, I will be eternally grateful.

On the Thursday evening I was to speak at a fancy dinner raising money for cancer research. I found myself sitting next to Uri Geller, the other "entertainer" for the evening. After my talk, as a gesture of appreciation, he took the dessertspoon out of my hand and stroked it gently. The spoon bent to 90 degrees on its own volition and I was left thinking that maybe Harry Potter did have something to offer.

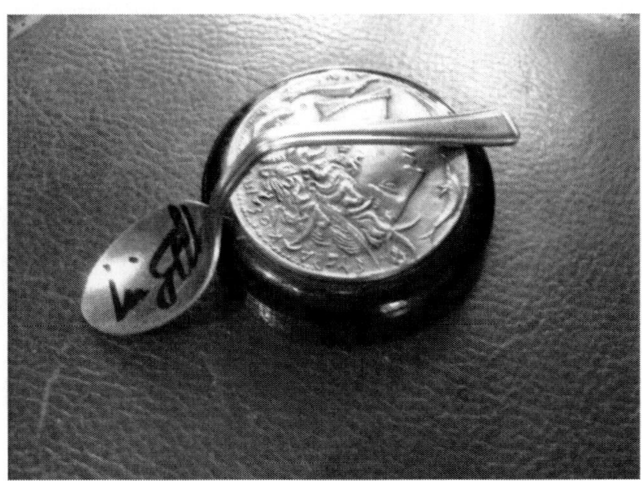

Bent spoon.

Fortunately my balance of mind was restored on Friday morning when I read Dominic Lawson's column in the Independent. His caption said it all:

"Can you tell the difference between homeopaths and witch doctors?"

"The answer is: witch doctors are not publicly funded within the NHS. Not so far, anyway."

Finally on Friday afternoon I took myself off to the British Museum to view the exhibition of Michelangelo's drawings. This is a wonderful journey into the transcendental. The centrepieces of the exhibition were his preparatory drawings for his master- work on the ceiling of the Sistine Chapel. What I had never realized before was that every image on that ceiling had been planned with exquisite care as a scaled down drawing. These drawings were scaled up using a matrix technique into full size cartoons all but one of which have been lost. The outlines on these cartoons were then transferred onto the wet plaster of segments of the roof for fresco painting by piercing the sheet with thousands of pin holes along the key lines and then rubbing in charcoal. The highlight of the exhibition for me was the interactive display whereby you could build up a fresco by selecting and transposing photographic segments from the original drawings that fitted in place like a jigsaw. This was evidence- based art (EBA) at its best. It doesn't save lives but it sure as hell saved my sanity.

Chapter 19

The Scam of Integrative Medicine

(Rapid response on line, BMJ 2011)

I've just returned from a delightful holiday with my American grandchildren in the Berkshires MA. The beautiful weather, the rolling hills, the pretty New England whitewashed houses and the Boston Symphony Orchestra playing in the open air at Tanglewood, all added to my sense of well being. I wish we could prescribe this regimen for our sick patients on the NHS.

Purely by chance I can offer an illustrative anecdote describing one of the hazards of so called integrative medicine that has so far been missed in the tsunami of rapid responses that greeted Margaret McCartney's message from the front line "The scam of integrative medicine". (BMJ 16th July, 343; 160, 2011)

We rented a lovely Victorian house near to Tanglewood and were rapidly shown round the facilities by a charming woman aged about 40 who was the owner, before being left to our own devices. I was curious to note a fridge magnet bearing the enigmatic words,

"Miso soup cures 50% of breast cancer says National Cancer Institute".

This associated with a cupboard full of vitamins, mineral food supplements and a concentrate of soya beans, allowed me put two and two together and deduce that, a) the owner was a victim of breast cancer and b) she was into alternative medicine in a big way. As our vacation came to an end and we were packed to go, the owner returned and engaged me in conversation. It didn't take long for her to figure out what I did for a living and she was anxious to share with me the good news about how she cured herself of breast cancer by the use of integrative medicine. She proudly told me about her 7 cm tumour and how she avoided surgery by putting together a team of experts that in addition to the local oncologist included a cancer nutritionist, who placed her on a macrobiotic diet, with plentiful supplements and a liquid concentrate of soy equivalent to 12lbs of the beans daily. She was also into meditation, Reiki and all the other usual suspects making up a team of six different "experts".

After three years she was on the point of giving up her only orthodox (read "evidence based") therapy, tamoxifen. Although how much value that might have been under the tidal wave of phyto-oestrogens she was imbibing, I couldn't begin to speculate. She had of course done the rounds of the orthodox medical specialities that included medical, surgical and radiation oncology and put together a complex regimen that she felt was tailored to her individual needs. I pleaded with her if nothing else, to carry on taking the tam.

Since coming home I checked on the NCI's recommendation for Miso soup and as might be expected it selectively referred to a publication in the JNCI from an observational study that suggested that a high intake of Miso soup might prevent breast cancer [1] although a more recent and methodologically sound study, could find no such an association [2].

So what does this story tell me? Firstly lay people and news headline writers are not adequately educated to interpret scientific disputations in scholarly journals or will be inclined to reinterpret or select published material, to support their pet prejudices. Secondly and perhaps of greater importance and greater hazard, is the relativism of "integrative medicine". If orthodox and alternative medicine are given equal weight and if the practitioners of evidence based medicine and unproven medicine are offered equal respect, then what's to stop patients like this to pick and mix to select the regimen of their choice in the name of person centred care? Perhaps Margaret, "scam" is too harsh a word as it implies evil intent when most of the advocates of alternative medicine are well meaning but naïve: Unless you were using SCAM as an acronym for Scandal of Complementary and Alternative Medicine.

References

[1] Yamamoto S, Sobue T, Kobayashi M, Sasaki S, Tsugane S; Japan Public Health Center-Based Prospective Study on Cancer and Cardiovascular Diseases Group. Soy, isoflavones, and breast cancer risk in Japan. *J Natl Cancer Inst* 2003;95:906–13.

[2] Nishio K, Niwa Y, Toyoshima H, Tamakoshi K, Kondo T, Yatsuya H, Yamamoto A, Suzuki S, Tokudome S, Lin Y, Wakai K, Hamajima N, Tamakoshi A. Consumption of soy foods and the risk of breast cancer: findings from the Japan Collaborative Cohort (JACC) Study. *Cancer Causes Control*. 2007 Oct;18(8):801-8.

Chapter 20

An Unusual Opportunity to Study the "Natural History" of Hormone Sensitive Breast Cancer

A friend of mine who is a Consultant Endocrinologist first referred IL to me in February 2005. She was 45 years old at the time and had become aware of a lump in the upper central part of right breast about three years prior to being seen. She had sought an opinion from a highly respected breast cancer specialist at that time but refused all investigations and treatment because she had the fixed belief, that invasive procedures would spread the cancer around the body and hasten her death. Instead she decided on taking homeopathy, vitamin and herbal supplements.

However she became aware that the tumour varied in size and discomfort according to the menstrual cycle and she herself deduced that the tumour was oestrogen dependent and that is why she went to see an endocrinologist before she came to my attention.

When I first met her, my initial impression that she would be something of a "weirdo" was not supported by the fact that she was personable, smartly dressed, intelligent and articulate.

On clinical examination the cancer had ulcerated through the skin over an area 2x2 cm and there was an underlying mass 6 x 6 cm in diameter with no deep fixation and no clinical evidence of regional lymphadenopathy. Once again I explained to her that the conventional approach would be to get a histological diagnosis with a core cut biopsy and then treat her with limited surgery, radiotherapy and appropriate systemic therapy. She listened to me politely and with respect but said she had made her own decisions and she would like me to treat her with some kind of endocrine manipulation.

I therefore started her with depot injections of goseralin 3.6mgs to suppress her ovarian function. Somewhat to my surprise she accepted my advice and attended my clinic on a regular basis, for me to personally provide the injections. Within a month the ulcer had begun to heal and was only 0.5cms in diameter and there was a measurable reduction in the diameter of the tumour. Within the passage of another month the ulcer had fully healed and the underlying tumour now measured 4 x 4cms. By the beginning of July the ulcer had completely healed and the tumour was reduced to 2.5cms maximum diameter. However a month later when she came for her sixth injection, I noticed that the tumour looked active again and that it was rather inflamed and oedematous. On this occasion she allowed me to perform the first diagnostic test, which was an ultrasound scan, which showed the obvious appearance of a carcinoma with a diameter of 4cms in size. I reiterated my original advice but still she demurred. On the pretty fair assumption that she was hormone receptor positive I had in mind to start her on an aromatase inhibitor to inhibit oestrogen production from the adrenal glands, but unfortunately when I saw her in September, things were getting worse and the ulcer was infected and beginning to haemorrhage. I then tried to persuade her to have radiotherapy but she has read of some promising results from cryosurgery only available in the island of Crete. When challenged as to why she would prefer such experimental treatment instead of the tried and tested approach of surgery and radiotherapy she advised me that radiotherapy can suppress immunity and surgery can stimulate the spread of cancer!

After the first course of cryotherapy combined with dressings of honey and herbs she came back to see me ecstatic that the cancer had “fallen off”. In fact all that had happened was that the ulcer had increased in size and the edges were necrotic. At that point she decided to go and live in Crete until she was cured and I haven’t heard from her again.

Chapter 21

A Letter to the Editor Declining a Book Review for Focus on Alternative and Complementary Therapy (FACT)

I'm not sure if the editor of FACT is playing an April fool trick on me by sending me this exercise in post-modern male ruminant excreta. If not, the fact remains that you will need to get another reviewer, as I have nothing printable to pass on to the authors. For a start I didn't understand what "natural therapists" were. Later on I discovered that they were the usual suspects practising alternative medicine. They also use and abuse words like "paradigm" and "holistic" without really understanding the meaning of the words. Their case is based on an assertion that "...in order to revert from ill health to wellness, patients need to understand why they are sick". Who says? In 40 years of clinical practice as a surgeon, oncologist and professor of medical humanities, I have returned thousands of patients to wellness without them having to understand microbiology or the genetics of malignant transformation. I've written three books to help my patients with this understanding but few have chosen to read my books. They are usually satisfied with my simple explanations in the clinic that include the rationale for treatment.

Things get worse when the authors assert "...patients can't make wise decisions if they are not informed properly". Yet they make it clear to me that the information provided by the "natural therapist" is false as for example when they take credit for explaining the philosophy of homeopathy. In other words their patients are not informed properly and are therefore encouraged to make foolish decisions.

I nearly gave up the will to live before reaching the end of the paper but I'm glad I read it through because I had a sudden flash of understanding. As alternative therapies, by definition are nothing but placebos, then the success of these interventions results from encouraging false concepts of the causality of disease that are easier to understand without a scientific education, than the truth.

Feel free to extract exerts from this to show to the authors but all in all I'd rather you found another referee who was not in the pocket of "big pharma" nor guilty of subscribing to the *western hegemony of the non-holistic bio-medical paradigm of inhumane doctrinaire high tech scientific medicine.*

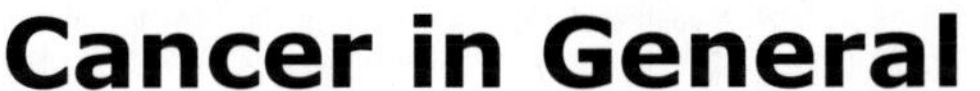
Cancer in General

Chapter 22

What Are the Needs of Patients Diagnosed with Cancer?

(Psycho-Oncology Volume 13, Issue 12, pages 850–852, December 2004)

I'm writing this piece in the lovely winter sunshine in Sydney where I am attending a cancer congress, having just learnt of the turbulence I've created in my open letter to HRH the Prince of Wales in the BMJ. [See http://www.bmj.com/content/329/7457/118]

I'm taking this opportunity to correct many of the misconceptions I've already picked up from the media feeding frenzy that tracked me down, down-under. Sharks I expected, but this! Most of my friends and professional colleagues have applauded the position I've taken but I am distressed by some of the hostile commentaries I've received in the BMJ rapid response columns, that seem to start with the premise that I'm a cold hearted bigot of an antiquated medical establishment. Below is my "manifesto" where I have drawn my lines in the sand, feel free to attack me by crossing these lines but not as a result of any misunderstanding of my position.

The Needs of Cancer Patients

Patients diagnosed with cancer have many needs. The diagnosis comes as a shock and maybe for the first time the individual is facing up to his or her mortality. So before we even think about the role of medicine we must consider their needs for moral and spiritual support. At times like this a close supportive family and membership of a faith community are invaluable and should not be "medicalized". Sadly there are many cancer sufferers who lack family support and in these secular days have no spiritual mentor. Such people may be drawn to "new age" belief groups in order to fill this aching void. If this provides some kind of spiritual solace I have no problem but if this is dressed up as "cure by magic" I draw the line.

The next need for the cancer subject is to be free of whatever symptoms plague their life as a result of the disease. Of course in the early stages the patients may be symptom free but in the later stages suffering from pain, nausea and weakness. Here we need collaboration by a team that includes doctors, nurses, and practitioners in professions that are complementary to medicine to help the patient feel better and improve the quality of life. The science of pain control is well established and palliative care for those close to the end is a well-developed specialty in the UK thanks to our hospice movement. Relatively new is the discipline of "Psycho-social oncology" which aims to identify and manage the more subtle subjective symptoms of cancer such as anxiety and depression. This field of activity really took off about 20 years ago with the development of psychometric instruments that could identify these often hidden problems. I chair the psychosocial oncology committee of our National Cancer Research Institute, which includes membership from our Consumer's group in addition to nurses, psychiatrists, psychologists and cancer clinicians. In this domain I believe there is a role for interventions such as therapeutic massage, acupuncture and counselling to help the patient feel better but again I draw the line at claims that these approaches alone can cure cancer. I concede that there exists a mind body nexus that in theory could be modulated to influence the natural course of the disease and through my committee am trying to encourage such research but at present I'm unaware of any reliable evidence that a psycho-somatic approach can replace proven medical therapy.

The third need of cancer victims is to be cured or at least have their lives prolonged. At this point a short digression is in order to consider a brief history of the subject. From the years 200 to 1800 CE, following the teachings of Aristotle and Galen, cancer was believed to be a consequence of the coagulation of "black bile" (melancholia) in the target organ. Black bile was one of the four metaphysical humours (black bile, yellow bile, phlegm and blood) that needed to be in balance for perfect health. The therapeutic responses to this belief were purgation (enemas), leaching, cupping (as exhibited by Gwyneth Paltrow's back last week) blood letting and extreme diets. Please note the similarity of this portfolio to popular alternative remedies of today. They didn't work and the patient's suffering was increased. In the last 200 years we have learnt much about the exquisite mechanisms of the body at molecular, cellular, whole organ and whole person levels. The realities are more beautiful, awesome and mysterious than ever dreamt of in Galen's philosophy.

In the late 19thC with the development of anaesthesia and antisepsis radical surgery began to replace irrational nostrums. Not long after this radiotherapy was introduced that increased the chances of local control of the cancer. These early successes in functional and symptomatic relief lead to a period of complacency in my profession which began to be shaken with the development of effective (albeit toxic) chemotherapy regimens and less toxic hormonal agents for hormone sensitive cancers such as those of the breast and prostate about 30 years ago. At the same time, the randomised controlled trial was introduced to critically evaluate combinations of these three modalities measuring both efficacy (improvement in survival) and tolerability. Using this approach we have made slow incremental improvements and can now negotiate with our patients "trade offs" between increasing length of life and the toxicity/ side effects of the treatments with a degree of precision and individualization that increases with each trial completed.

In my own subject, breast cancer, the last 20 years has shown remarkable progress. Having inherited the radical mastectomy as therapeutic dogma we can now safely offer breast preservation without compromising cure whilst the addition of drugs tailored to the biology of the disease has contributed to a 30% reduction in mortality.

20 years ago I wrote an article in the Evening Standard in response to the challenge of HRH the Prince of Wales to the BMA on its 150th anniversary.

Yes the profession has been complacent in the past in ignoring the humanitarian aspects of medicine but that has changed and the "humanities" are now central to our undergraduate curriculum but of equal importance is the evaluation of evidence. Modern medicine is now evidence based and being practiced with increasing humanity. The proponents of alternative medicine do not have a monopoly on compassion and empathy and the promotion of unproven therapies or the diversion of scarce resources from rational treatment to the practices popular in the dark ages, is unlikely to contribute greatly in reducing the sum of human suffering.

Chapter 23

Scientific Method and the Search for the Cure for Cancer

"Blue-Sky Cancer Research" Cambridge 2000

All great painters failed to be recognized in their lifetime. I'm a painter who has not been recognized in his lifetime therefore I'm great. In fact I *am* a painter, a gifted amateur, but with sufficient insight to know that I will never amount to much. The assertion in the first sentence is known as a syllogism and is a well-recognized error in logic. The same logical trap neatly describes the history of science. I have just finished reading the hugely entertaining book, "A short history of nearly everything" by Bill Bryson. In this book he traces the history of the great discoveries in cosmology, geology, palaeontology and life science. Within this book he celebrates the giants and geniuses of scientific ideas since the age of enlightenment. It is certainly true that progress was often dependant on the revolutionaries who challenged the prevailing dogma and were in return ridiculed and often dying in obscurity, before the main stream accepted their ideas. Major shifts in our understanding of nature and the cosmos resulted from the overturning of the conceptual model of the problem rather than the accumulation of "facts". But beware, it does not follow that all revolutionaries who are prepared to challenge the prevailing dogma are great scientists. The book that describes the other side of this coin is called "Voodoo science" by Robert Park, equally entertaining but sounding a cautionary note. Some self-appointed scientific revolutionaries can be both mad and bad!

In mid winter 2000, I chaired a meeting at Cambridge University, which was entitled "Blue sky-cancer research". The meeting was funded by a group of merchant bankers and the invitees came from every walk of life. There was an inner circle of clinical and basic scientists and an outer circle of representatives from finance, economics, politics, philosophy and the arts. We all had two things in common- frustration with the pace of progress in cancer research and a willingness to think "outside the box". Many exciting ideas emerged from a long weekend of brainstorming and a road map for blue-sky research was proposed which not surprisingly failed to find financial backers from either the research councils or business. Perhaps some of the ideas were a bit wacky but all those who attended and signed up to this portfolio of ideas were high achievers in their own fields so as a group at least we weren't all mad and bad.

All the rhetoric concerning cancer treatment and cancer research is couched in the terms of military conflict. The politicians trumpet the fact that we are winning the war against cancer. We talk about mobilising resources and the cancer researchers with the highest public profile are described in terms, normally reserved for military leaders. At the sharp end the poor patient never simply dies of the disease but loses the fight. This terminology fixes in the mind of the public and the politicians the idea that cancer is a foreign invader and therefore the war against cancer is aimed at destroying every last malignant cell.

This is a false analogy. The cancer cells are simply an undisciplined sub-stratum of our own cells. Cancer is an inevitable component of the aging process and all of us at some time in our lives co-exist with latent cancer scattered around the body. No wonder the most aggressive modern treatments can end up killing the person, before killing the cancer. Medical oncologist often complain about the narrow therapeutic ratio within which they have to work—in other words the differences between the normal cell and the cancer cell are so small that they can rarely be exploited to the patients' benefit. No, we are not winning the war against cancer and the aggregate mortality for malignant disease has barely changed since President Nixon declared war in 1971.

In 1971 President Nixon launched his war against cancer with the now notorious Cancer Act. In the same way President Kennedy, had promised to land a man on the moon in the 1960's, so Nixon would find a cure for cancer in the 1970's. I was working in Pittsburgh with Professor Bernard Fisher at the time and shared his deep scepticism about the possibility to deliver on this promise. When Kennedy promised the Americans that they would land a man on the moon we knew with a very high degree of accuracy where the target lay. All that remained was to create the technology based on the rocketry developed in the Second World War. By comparison, for cancer, we did not know in 1971 where the target was and the conventional non-specific cytotoxic therapies were equivalent to firing off rockets in random directions.

Undoubtedly there have been dramatic breakthroughs in the treatments of leukaemia, lymphoma and the childhood cancers. Thirty years ago all these would have been fatal but today we can expect between 50% and 75% cure rates (depending on subtypes). These followed on from the classic experiments with animal models and cytotoxic chemotherapy in the 1960s and as it turns out this group of diseases are exquisitely sensitive to cytotoxic drugs. Unfortunately the very diseases that are most responsive to chemotherapy tend to be extremely rare and count for less than 5% of the total cancer burden. Furthermore the very success of chemotherapy in these rare cancers has paradoxically delayed progress in discovering effective treatments for the more common solid tumours such as colorectal and bronchogenic carcinoma that have stubbornly refused to respond in significant numbers to these very toxic treatments. Instead of the *reductio ad absurdum* of persisting with high dose chemotherapy to virtually lethal doses, we should try to learn from mistakes of the past and understand why rare cancers respond to chemotherapy but common cancers do not. All that aside, what else of importance can be learnt from trends in incidence and mortality? The incidence of some cancers falls or rises for reasons that are not understood. For example at one extreme, stomach cancer, which is very common in Japan, is rapidly disappearing in the west. We now have a generation of young surgeons who have never cut their teeth on a radical gastrectomy for this horrid disease. There must be lifestyle reasons or environmental changes to explain what has happened but these are still a mystery. At the other extreme, malignant myeloma (a malignant process effecting the bone marrow) is increasing worldwide, almost as if there had been a viral vector.

In contrast however the trends in the incidence of lung cancer and along with this lung cancer mortality are easy to explain. In Britain and the US lung cancer mortality for men fell rapidly once there was a clearly established link between smoking and the disease. Tragically many young women are now taking up the habit, as a result of which deaths from lung cancer have overtaken deaths from breast cancer amongst women in North America and Britain. There is only one of the common cancers that can truly be viewed as a success story of modern treatment—that is breast cancer where treatment has contributed to about a 30% reduction in mortality over the last 15 years. This can largely be ascribed to the fact that breast cancer, unlike the majority of other cancers, is peculiarly sensitive to the level of sex hormones in the circulation and we now have safe and effective drugs that can modify these oestrogen levels. But as far as the other common cancers are concerned—lung cancer, bowel cancer, cancer of the ovary, cancer of the cervix, cancer of the prostate—little in the way of therapeutic advances have been seen in spite of the billions of dollars thrown into cancer research and treatment since Nixon's initiative of 30 years ago.

Let us now consider the received wisdom about cancer that mark out the conceptual constraints, which determine all programmes of fundamental research into the problem.

Cancer is a molecular problem. Either by inheritance or by exogenous factors that target us through life, specific cells accumulate sufficient mutations that have escaped natural DNA repair mechanisms to exhibit the properties of a malignant phenotype. The cancer cell then has the capacity for promiscuous growth, immortality, infiltration, dissemination and the establishment of remote colonies. The cancer then kills by unrestrained growth in a closed compartment e.g. brain tumours or by their metastases that destroy vital organs such as the liver, lung or bone marrow. The triumphalistic reception to the news that the human genome had been decoded, with President Bush and Prime Minister Tony Blair standing side by side in front of banks of cameras to announce the news, was fuelled in part by the assumption that the complete understanding and cure of cancer was just around the corner. Sadly unlike the war in Iraq the war against cancer is still being lost. I don't wish to minimalise the achievement of cracking the code; it is indeed a triumph of human ingenuity, technology and perseverance. Unfortunately there are even taller mountains to conquer before we can begin to understand the cancer cell and its relationship with the host's body. It is common parlance to talk about the tumour/ host relationship yet that is a give-away, disclosing the assumption that the cancer cell is an alien parasite. In fact one of the problems in treating cancer is the similarity of the cancer to its progenitors and the plasticity of the cancer cell, with its capacity to re-differentiate to a normal cell or even another fully differentiated adult phenotype.

The genetic code merely reads off the instructions for lining up the amino acids in the appropriate sequence for a specific protein. This string of amino acids then has to fold into exotic shapes before the protein can function. The understanding of how the folds are determined and how the three-dimensional shape determines function is known as proteomics and this is the next great challenge. But even that is barely scratching at the surface of the awesome task of understanding how tens of thousands of these complex molecules interact with each other to create a cell and how millions of cells interact with each other to create you and me. Only then when we have recreated the human subject from the rubble of molecular reductionism will we have a glimmer of understanding of how the fault in the gene or the fault in the folding of a protein or the fault in the cross talk or geometry of cell to cell interaction leads to the human suffering of cancer. Imagine the task of rebuilding a functioning Boeing 747 from the scattered components of a deconstructed plane without a blueprint and a less than complete understanding of the physics of flight, amplify that challenge a million times and that gives you feel of the magnitude of the task ahead. But then pause for a moment and consider that the genetic abnormalities of cancer may not be the direct cause of the malignant transformation but in part an indirect consequence of faults at different levels in the hierarchical organization of the body just described, feeding back to destabilize the human genome. If that is the case then much of the current programme of cancer research is misdirected. It reminds me of the story of the drunk trying to find the key to his house under a lamppost some distance from his front door. When challenged on this, he declared with hurt dignity that this was where there was sufficient light to see the key. The techniques of molecular biology certainly shine sufficient light but maybe the key to cancer is in the penumbra of that zone.

I'm often surprised by the hostility of the response when I politely challenge a speaker at a scientific conference on the assumptions that underpin his favourite hypothesis. We are sometimes wedded to our ideas with greater fidelity than we are wedded to our wives. As Thomas Huxley once stated-"The great tragedy of science is the slaying of a beautiful hypothesis by an ugly fact". I believe there are now so many outlying facts that we are at a point of crisis with the molecular paradigm of cancer. But simply wrecking a paradigm is not sufficient; we need a new set of beliefs that can explain the successes of the past yet incorporate all the outlying facts that spoil the picture.

For a start I think that we need to look at the new mathematics of non-linear systems and consider how one of the stigmata of cancer is the loss of the perfect fractal geometry of duct and vascular systems. If we consider the breast in women, the prostate in men and the thyroid in both sexes, then all of us at most times carry latent (usually referred to as in-situ) cancers. They demonstrate loss of heterozygosity, evidence of genetic mutations. However only a minority of such lesions progress to invasive cancer otherwise all of us would die of the disease. However if we consider these as a necessary but not sufficient condition for cancer then we can develop a beautiful model of carcinogenesis that can incorporate most of the outlying observations.

To avoid duplication I now turn your attention to section 27.

Chapter 24

Prevention Is Better Than Cure! I Wouldn't Be So Sure Mr. Brown

(Spiked 14th Jan 2008)

On Monday the 7th of January 2008, Prime Minister Gordon Brown launched a new NHS initiative in public health policy by repeating that wearisome cliché; "prevention is better than cure". This was followed by announcing a raft of screening initiatives aimed at achieving immortality for all, which seemed to take the medical profession by surprise. Who, if anyone, had been consulted?

I have served the NHS loyally for over 40 years and I feel that I deserve a campaign medal for every reorganization or new initiative I've faced, taken by governments of all political hues, but this latest one I regard as Nature's way of telling me to resign my commission without facing another battle.

So by way of a swansong let me explain to our prime minister, whose political party my family has actively supported through three generations, why he might just want to take further advice on these new proposals.

First of all, screening is not prevention of disease but detection of asymptomatic disease. Screening theory has it, that the detection of the earliest stages of a disease before it creates symptoms followed by prompt treatment might postpone death; but of course not prevent death. Death is inevitable like taxes and NHS reorganizations. Prevention literally means avoiding the onset of a specific disease and presupposes that we fully understand the aetiology of the disease in question. However the fundamental problem with both the prevention of disease and the early asymptomatic diagnosis of disease is that the whole population is exposed to an intervention and its unwelcome side effects, for the benefit of a minority. In contrast, cure of a disease, is targeted at the individual who reaps the benefits and "pays the price". By "paying the price" I'm talking about inconvenience and toxic side effects rather than cash up front.

In the practice of bedside medicine there is an ethical imperative of autonomy and informed consent. As a surgeon and an oncologist I have to inform the patient of the benefits versus the harms of my intervention whether it's by surgery or the prescription of drugs. With the expansion of evidence-based medicine (EBM) in oncology, we can do this with increasing precision and individualization. With the practice of public health interventions of screening and prevention the evidence base tends be less robust and the ethical model of respect for autonomy very poorly developed.

At one extreme of course, advice on healthy lifestyles that include the avoidance of tobacco products, regular modest exercise, plenty of fruit and vegetables and a little red wine, can indeed extend life expectancy [1] and enhance quality of life with little in the way of toxic side effects. Providing the government don't become all sanctimonious about this, with thought police, exercise police, diet police, smoking police and withholding health care for "self inflicted" sickness, I have no problem with promoting such good advice. The problem though becomes much more difficult when the intervention is a test or a "treatment", or a "treatment" as the consequence of a test.

Before we can sanction these kinds of interventions we must have robust evidence from randomized controlled trials of large and representative populations that the test or the treatment can reduce mortality from the disease with a favourable benefit/harm ratio, that is explicitly stated, to satisfy individual choice. In addition we need to be confident that the opportunity costs of such a programme don't consume too many resources as to threaten the funding for treatment and cure of symptomatic disease. These are not the words of some maverick but can be taken as a summary of an excellent book, "Screening, Evidence and Practice", by Angela Raffle, Consultant in Public Health and the National screening programmes and Sir Muir Gray, Programmes Director of the UK National Screening Committee 1996-2007. [2]

"Whereof one cannot speak, thereof one must be silent" stated Wittgenstein. Quite so Ludwig, but I can speak with authority about my own health and also about breast cancer.

To start with, my first hand experience can inform and illustrate the debate very nicely, as it describes the best of preventative action already available in the NHS, long before the Prime Minister's announcement. My youngest brother David died of a massive heart attack at the age of 59 whilst in office as President of the Royal College of Paediatrics and Child Health. After a period in mourning I took myself off to see my local GP, Dr. Chris Page, who counselled me on the harms and benefits of screening for ***risk*** of heart disease. He explained a risk assessment model factoring in family history, blood pressure, smoking history and blood lipid levels. He went on to explain how for each increasing increment of risk there were interventions of known toxicity that could modify this risk by a measurable quantity that could be described in absolute numbers rather than relative risk reductions. (See later) All of this was illustrated by coloured, decision aid diagrams. I came to a well-informed decision that it would be in my best interest to have my blood pressure monitored and my serum lipids measured. (Smoking advice was not required as I'd never started.) My BP was mildly elevated as was my total cholesterol. For the last two years I've been taking statins and a mild diuretic without toxic side effects. For this inconvenience I've perhaps reduced my risk of a myocardial infarct by about 1 in 10. [3] This experience illustrates the best of evidence-based prevention within the NHS. I now wish to compare this with my knowledge of what's on offer for women by way of prevention and screening for breast cancer.

Most of my career has been devoted to the research and treatment of breast cancer and I have been in the front line in the development of screening and prevention of the disease. Furthermore my family has been afflicted with breast cancer making the challenge up front and personal. [4]

Let's start with prevention. Most of the risk factors are beyond our control i.e. sex, age, race and genetic inheritance. Some risk reduction might be possible by adopting the healthy life style behaviours described above [1] together with the avoidance of binge drinking and if there is a choice in the matter, starting a family before the age of 30. However we are still searching for the holy grail of chemoprevention of breast cancer. In 1985 Jack Cuzick and I published a very important observation in the Lancet [5], describing how women, with breast cancer, treated with adjuvant tamoxifen demonstrated a significant reduction in the risk of a new breast cancer of the other breast. This observation was confirmed by other studies and led to the launch of the IBIS 1 trial for the prevention of breast cancer with tamoxifen amongst women at a high risk. This and similar trials confirmed that tamoxifen could lead to a relative risk reduction (RRR) in the incidence of breast cancer by more than

30% at the cost of some significant side effects. [6] This study provides an excellent example on how to calculate benefit/harm analyses that might inform public policy and allow the individual subject to judges for themselves.

For a start let me try and explain relative risk reduction.

Most statisticians and epidemiologists describe risks in relative terms such as 50% increase or 25% reduction. To translate this into simple numbers demands an understanding of the background risk. Let me provide a simple illustration. Say a young student is involved in fieldwork in Siberia and is keen to come home for Christmas but only has £300 to spend on airfares. A flight on BA would cost £500 but a flight on Air Uzbluchistan (AU) is within his budget. Just before he travels he learns that AU has a less that perfect safety record with a 50% increase in the chance of crashing compared with BA. To understand that risk, that sounds very alarming he needs to know BA safety record. He then learns that BA only crashes one in every 2,000,000 flights (i.e. risk is 0.000002%) a 50% increase in that risk is an extra 1:1,000,000 (i.e. an absolute risk of 0.000003%).

He can then judge whether he can accept that risk and will probably fly. In other words a 50% increase of a very small risk maybe a risk worth taking and the reverse is also true, that a 50% decrease of a very small risk is a very small gain.

Now let's compute the absolute benefits of chemoprevention of breast cancer.

The normal risk for women is about 2:1,000 a year. The women in IBIS 1 had a background risk of about 3 times that, 6:1,000 a year or 6% in a decade. A 30%RRR would mean that about 2% might avoid breast cancer over a decade at the cost of increased hazard of thrombosis, endometrial cancer and other gynaecological problems. [6] In the USA it is commonplace to accept this trade off but as for myself, a co-author of the study, I don't think the gain is worth the pain. Yet we still continue the search. The IBIS 2 trial is of a similar design but instead of using tamoxifen is using the aromatase inhibitor, anastrozole, which has been shown to be twice as effective as tamoxifen in preventing contralateral breast cancer with a much better safety profile. [7]

Who knows, that might be a preventative with a sufficient benefit harm ratio to win over the informed woman at increased risk of breast cancer.

Now let us adopt the same principle for mammographic screening for breast cancer.

Proponents of screening, often parade women who claim that, "screening saved their life". Most lay-people and screening zealots think that is the killer argument, well in a way it is. It kills off the debate at a stroke, not because it can't be rebutted but because people like me find it difficult to be unkind. I believe the time is long past when we have to patronize womenfolk in order to retain our popularity.

Every woman can interpret her screening experience in a way that reinforces her decision to accept the invitation. The result was negative; thank God for the reassurance. The result was a false alarm; well you can't be too careful.

The result showed duct carcinoma in situ (DCIS); thank God it was caught before it had a chance to spread. The result showed invasive cancer; thank God it was caught early.

Let us now re-examine those four scenarios.

Just how much reassurance is a negative result worth? For a start most women overestimate their risk of developing breast cancer. [8] If we stick with post-menopausal women, then the annual risk of developing breast cancer in a normal population is 2:1,000 a year and say, as in the UK, screening is at three yearly intervals then the accumulated risk over three years is 6:1,000. Therefore in each period 994:1,000 women might expect **not** to develop the disease. Assuming that the interval cancer rate (i.e. those cancers that develop between the first and second round of screening) is about a third of the screen detected rate, [9] then only an additional 4:1,000 woman over three years win extra reassurance.

In the second scenario no woman has a gain. It's like thanking the fireman for rescuing you from the fire when he threw you in to begin with! This false alarm and unnecessary surgery is of no value to the woman. It can even be damaging in a subtle way, if as a chance finding the benign nodule or scar is close to an area of atypical ductal hyperlasia (ADH) or in situ lobular carcinoma, which then classifies the woman as at an increased risk, and then what does she do apart from worry?

The third scenario follows the detection of duct carcinoma DCIS. In about 30%-40% of such cases the disease is multi-focal and the woman is advised mastectomy for this "early" breast cancer. [10] Yet if left undetected some might regress and others might co-exist with the woman for the rest of her life. [11] Whenever a screening programme starts, 20% of the screen-detected cancers are DCIS and screening theory would suggest that their detection would ultimately lead to a fall in invasive cancers in the population. Not so; there is also a long- term **increase** in the incidence of invasive cancers. [12, 13].

Finally the third scenario; yes indeed a life might have been saved. As I have described and as also backed up by many others [14,15], the estimate of number of lives saved is about 1:1,000 per10 years of screening. (Note this is two orders of magnitude less than the benefits I described for the prevention of heart disease). Yet it does not follow that the screen detection of each cancer represents a life saved. If left to nature the cancer might have progressed slowly, became clinically obvious and cured by treatment on presentation. After all we are close to curing 75% of cases with modern therapy [16] and screening is good at detecting "good" cancers. It's the bad cancers that slip through the net and appear as interval cases. [17] Furthermore, some of the cancers are so slow growing that if undetected would never appear in a woman's lifetime. These are what Welch describes as pseudo-cancers. [18] Last of all, we never know for sure if indeed a life has been saved when mammography detects a cancer. A small grade III cancer even if node negative has a lethal capacity even if caught "early". The biology of a tumour is more important than its chronology.

For too long the mantra of screening, "catch it early and we will save your life and save your breast", has been allowed to go unchallenged. Breast cancer is too complex a problem for such a facile solution. For too long women have been patronized and coerced into screening. And now the government want to extend the age for screening below the age of 50 in the face of the recently published UK trial that showed no significant advantage for this age group. [19]

Conclusion

I trust that the department of health will learn from the errors of the past and not be rushed into programmes of screening for prostate cancer, bowel cancer, ovarian cancer and other pathologies without having evidence based harm/benefit analyses to offer the individual to allow them to make an informed choice. If they decide no thank you, so be it. In discussing the ethical issues of screening we must accept a tension that exists between "Utilitarian" principles and those of "Autonomy". Utilitarianism involves social engineering for the "greatest good of the greatest number", whereas autonomy assumes the individual has an informed choice when health interventions for "their own good" are considered. Social engineering and coercion might be acceptable for hygiene and substance abuse, but when the balance of benefit versus harm is a close call then surely the right to self -determination trumps the principle of utilitarianism? Nowhere is this truer than in the area of screening for cancer. We screen for cancer to reduce cause-specific mortality without an increase in all cause mortality and at an acceptable cost in terms of medical morbidity. Even where their is level one evidence from RCTs of a reduction in cancer specific mortality, the benefit in absolute risk reduction maybe so small that the individual should have the right to make a personal trade off against the undoubted harms of false alarms, over-diagnosis and radical treatments for diseases that, if left to nature, would never announce themselves in a lifetime. I therefore propose that the uncritical promotion of screening is unethical by modern ethical standards and reflects a paternalistic attitude that would be unacceptable for treatment aimed at curing established disease. In these cases cure is better than prevention.

References

[1] Khaw KT, Wareham N, Bingham S, Welch A, Luben R, Day N Combined Impact of Health Behaviours and Mortality in Men and Women: The EPIC-Norfolk Prospective Population Study. *PLoS Med.* 2008 Jan 8;5(1):e12 [Epub ahead of print]

[2] Screening Evidence and Practice. Angela Raffle and Muir Gray, Oxford University Press, Oxford 2007.

[3] Fidan D, Unal B, Critchley J, Capewell S. Economic analysis of treatments reducing coronary heart disease mortality in England and Wales, 2000-2010.*QJM.* 2007 May;100(5):277-89.

[4] Baum M A lifetime in breast cancer research. *Eur J Cancer.* 2007 Jul;43(10):1496-7.

[5] Cuzick J, Baum M. Tamoxifen and contralateral breast cancer. *Lancet* 1985;ii:282.

[6] Cuzick, J., Forbes, J., Edwards, R., Baum, M., Cawthorn, S., Coates, A., et al., First results from the International Breast Cancer Intervention Study (IBIS-I): a randomised prevention trial. *Lancet*, 2002. 360(9336): p. 817-24.

[7] Howell, A., Cuzick, J., Baum, M., et al., Results of the ATAC (Arimidex, Tamoxifen, Alone or in Combination) trial after completion of 5 years' adjuvant treatment for breast cancer. *Lancet,* 2005. 365(9453): p. 60-2.

[8] Black W.C., Nease R.F. Jr., Tosteson A.N. Perceptions of breast cancer risk and screening effectiveness in women younger than 50 years of age. *Journal of the National Cancer Institute* 1995;87:720-731.

[9] Blanks RG, Moss SM, McGahan CE, Quinn MJ, Babb PJ. Effect of NHS breast screening programme on mortality from breast cancer in England and Wales, 1990-8: Comparison of observed with predicted mortality. *BMJ* 2000; 321:665-9.

[10] NHS cancer screening programmes. NHS Breast Screening Programme & British Association of Surgical Oncology Breast Group. An audit of screen detected breast cancers for the year of screening April 1999 to March 2000.16-5-2001.

[11] Collins LC, Tamimi RM, Baer HJ, Connolly JL, Colditz GA, Schnitt SJ Cancer. Outcome of patients with ductal carcinoma in situ untreated after diagnostic biopsy. *Cancer* 2005 May 1;103(9):1778-84.

[12] Zackrisson S, Andersson I, Manjer J and Garne JP, Rate of over-diagnosis of breast cancer 15 years after end of Malmö mammographic screening trial: follow up study. *BMJ* 2006;332:689-92.

[13] Møller H, Davies E, Over-diagnosis in breast cancer screening. *BMJ* 2006; 332: 691-692.

[14] Miller AB. The costs and benefits of breast cancer screening. *Am J Prev Med* 1993;9:175-80.

[15] Sarfati D. Howden-Chapman P. Woodward A. Salmond C. Does the frame affect the picture? A study into how attitudes to screening for cancer care are affected by the way benefits are expressed. *Journal of Medical Screening* 1998; 5(3):137-140.

[16] Vervoort MM, Draisma G, Frachebaud J, van de Poll-Franse, de koning HJ (2004). Trends in the usage of adjuvant systemic therapy for breast cancer in the Netherlands and its effect on mortality. *Br J Cancer* 91: 241-247.

[17] Watmough D.J. [1993] Interval Breast Cancers. *American J Roentgenology July* 1993, 161, 3.

[18] H.Gilbert Welch, "Should I be tested for Cancer?" University of California Press, 2004, ISBN 0520239768.

[19] Moss SM, Cuckle H, Evans A, Johns L, Waller M, Bobrow L, for the Trial Management Group. Effect of mammographic screening from age 40 years on breast cancer mortality at 10 years' follow-up: a randomised controlled trial. *Lancet* 2006;368:2053-60.

Chapter 25

Book Review for Spiked: The Secret War on Cancer

Devra Davis

(Spiked review of books March 2008)

I started reading this book on a flight to Stockholm. For light relief I bought the airport edition of John Grisham's new novel, "The Appeal". One book is a semi-fictional account of evil petrochemical firms poisoning the environment and causing cancer, with a political and legal conspiracy to hide the facts. And by amazing coincidence so was Grisham's novel! I'll give you two guesses as to which was the more readable.

The thesis in Devra Davis' secret war book runs as follows: The majority of cancers today are caused by environmental pollutants and there is a conspiracy of the biggest industrial companies in the USA, aided and abetted by government agencies and "hired guns" amongst the scientific establishment, to bury these facts along with the landfills of toxic effluent.

Devra Davis, PhD, MPH, is director of the Centre for Environmental Oncology at the University of Pittsburgh Cancer Institute. To begin with I was well disposed to her, as we seemed to have much in common. She makes much of her Jewish roots and how these traditions influenced her philosophy.

So do I.

I spent a seminal year in Pittsburgh working with the doyen of breast cancer research, Dr. Bernie Fisher, in 1971. I was there when Dr. Fisher co-signed the Nixon Cancer act, promising to find the cure for cancer in the 70s. Nixon wanted to upstage Kennedy when the American space agency, NASA, landed a man on the moon, during his administration. Dr. Fisher and I shared Dr. Davis' scepticism at this initiative. Nixon actually brought in NASA engineers to design a 10 year programme of R&D, based on the lunar landing project to lick cancer during his administration and also perhaps to deflect criticism about the US preoccupations in SE Asia. I clearly remember sharing the joke with Dr. Fisher as we gazed at a wall covered with flow charts and tick boxes that appeared to provide a road map to direct the cancer scientist to the Holy Grail.

Fisher was happy to take his share of the loot to follow his own line of research that eventually led to a 30% reduction in breast cancer mortality over the last 25 years. Our scepticism was based on understanding the difference between cosmology and oncology. We knew precisely where the moon was (next door in cosmological terms); we had rockets that could reach that far; so the rest was technology and engineering. We didn't know where cancer was in the 1970s, other than it was hiding somewhere in the vast micro cosmos of the cell. Sending off missiles at random (e.g. non specific chemotherapy) was as likely to miss the target and kill the patient as to contribute to a cure.

Dr. Davis' scepticism was based on the fact that nowhere in this vast wall chart was there a box to tick concerning the prevention of cancer from environmental carcinogens. Whilst I would agree immediately that this was a grave omission she goes further in claiming that excluding environmental pollutants is the complete answer to the cancer problem. She knows this for certain and will brook no argument. At this point she began to lose my sympathy. She seems to have abandoned the discomfort that most scientists experience in living with uncertainty and this book ends up as an evangelical polemic written in a tiresomely hectoring tone. What's even worse is when she pauses in lecturing us in order to introduce some folksy anecdotes that she offers up as proof of her prejudices of the same value as the formal epidemiological studies she selectively cites.

Epidemiology is something of a blunt instrument, very good at demonstrating associations but rather poor at demonstrating causality. Let me illustrate this by proving that the cathode ray tube causes breast cancer. There is a direct association between the ownership of TVs and the incidence of breast cancer. There are geographical differences in the incidence of breast cancer and the ownership of TVs. There is a dose response in that the more TVs per household the greater the incidence of breast cancer. Finally, in the Western world there has been a sudden increase in the incidence of breast cancer as the old cathode ray TVs are dumped in landfills, polluting the environment, as we moved over to the new flat screen monitors. Pretty convincing you have to agree. However there is another way of looking at it. TV ownership is a surrogate measure for the prosperity of a country. Prosperous women may delay their first pregnancy, become fat and indolent and drink too much wine. All of which are known to be risk factors for breast cancer. As for the flat screens-well they were introduced gradually at the same time programmes of mammographic screening for breast cancer were being rolled out in Europe.

Screening leads to the over-diagnosis of breast cancer and a sudden increase in incidence of close on 20%. After that cautionary note let me give examples of the good, the bad and the ugly components of this seriously flawed book.

When she's good, she's very very good. The second chapter on the history of epidemiology and the discovery of industrial diseases from scrotal cancer amongst chimney sweeps, cancers amongst the pioneers in the discovery of ionizing radiation and hydrocarbon carcinogenesis amongst the petroleum workers in the 1920s and 1930s is captivating. Marie Curie died of cancer and I'm one of the privileged few who have been allowed a short exposure to her laboratory at the Institut Curie in Paris. Her notebooks are still dangerously radioactive.

The third chapter on the work of the Nazi scientists is fascinating. There is no doubt they understood the hazards of tobacco and try to ban it in the name of hygiene for the Aryan race. There may indeed have been blindness to their work, because of its origins and some of the unsavoury experiments that underpinned their research. I think it was unlikely that there was a formal conspiracy of the allies to hide these data. Her long discussion on Nazi eugenics, although truly interesting and hateful, seems out of place in this book. On principle everything the Nazis were for: e.g. racial hygiene, organic farming, natural remedies, homeopathy and anti-vivisection, I'm against. Maybe I need to look again at the anti-tobacco campaigns, which are almost fascistic in their torment of the poor old guys addicted to the weed because of its still legal status. Chapters 4, 5, 7 and 12 are where she gets into her stride when she describes the history of the chemical industry, the tobacco industry and the asbestos manufacturers and their malignant fall out. Here there is little doubt that throughout the first 60 years or so of the 20thC there was a determined effort of industry to hide the evidence supporting the malignant potential of their products. 100% of workers in the benzidine dye workers of I.G.Farben developed bladder cancer after 25 years exposure in the 1930s, but this only appeared in the public domain in 1946. This was a shameful period in the history of industrialization and the development of the consumer society. A point of farce was reached when the tobacco giant manufacturing Lucky Strike, developed a "safer cigarette" by incorporating an asbestos filter tip! Davis makes a good point here in that the tobacco industry wanted it both ways, whilst vehemently denying the carcinogenic properties of their products and spent a fortune on trying to develop a safe alternative. The head of the National Cancer Institute, Kenneth Endicott, who was himself a chain smoker, supported this work.

Now to the bad: I could have chosen several chapters but the one that made me most angry, chapter 15 "presumed innocent", concerned amongst other things her unsubstantiated conviction that mobile phones cause brain cancer. "Why are more children developing cancer and learning problems?" she asks. Well actually they're not. "Why does the government of England advise that persons under 18 should not use mobile phones at all?" she asks again. Well they don't. In fact we are about to buy our 11-year old grand daughter one when she goes to her secondary school later this year. She describes the largest study of its kind, published by the Danish Cancer Society, which concluded there was no link between mobile phones and brain tumours- only to rubbish it. They failed to account for electromagnetic rays in coffee shops, they only looked at ten years of usage and the killer argument; they received funding from the telecommunication industry. She even claims that electromagnetic radiation causes male breast cancer by quoting relative risks that are not significant. Some of the other statistical manipulations she uses to advance her case against all the available evidence might be considered scientific misconduct if published in a peer reviewed journal. She ends up concluding that almost every aspect of modern life is a cause of cancer until proved otherwise. And yet, and yet, we who are privileged to live in the Westernized industrial nations are enjoying the longest expectation of life on record.

Finally the ugly: Every study that reinforces her prejudice is described as stunning and its authors described as distinguished. Every one that goes against her belief system is flawed and published by someone of no account.

She even describes R.A. Fisher as an ***obscure*** British statistician because she didn't like his results. Obscure! He was one of the most famous, with the eponymous "Fisher's exact test" and a blue plaque on the wall where he lived not far from my house. Worst of all though is the way she deals with Sir Richard Doll. Clearly she didn't see eye to eye with him on many issues but could hardly dismiss him as obscure. Along with Bradford Hill and Archie

Cochrane he was the greatest of the epidemiologists of the latter half of the last century. So she sets out to assassinate his character. On page 311 she writes, "We will probably never know whether Doll's ideas about how scientists should study industrial hazards were at all coloured by the fact that he secretly served as a highly paid consultant for the asbestos, chemical and pesticide industries." Well sadly Richard Doll is no longer here to defend himself as he died at the age of 94 just over a year ago. Like many in the British oncology community I knew Sir Richard and admired him enormously. I served on a number of data monitoring and safety committees under his chairmanship. He was a man of great principle, scientific integrity, modesty and charm. More than most of his generation along with my good friend Sir Richard Peto, he contributed to the massive fall in deaths from lung cancer in the last 30 years; the greatest success of all time in tackling the dangers of environmental pollution. He lived modestly in college at Oxford University and was the last one you could imagine taking backhanders.

I finished this book on a visit to Florence. After my lecture I went to visit the Palatine galleries of the Pitti Palace. The walls of the gallery are filled three rows high and five rows across with histrionic paintings clamouring for your attention. Yet unbidden, in each room, my attention was drawn to the sublime and peaceful paintings of the Madonna and child by Raphael. Their truth was manifest in spite of the background noise. That's how I feel about this book. Some of the chapters are masterpieces when she allows the facts to speak for themselves but the totality is seriously flawed by her shrillness and self-interested manipulation of the facts. One wonders whether the publisher ever employs an editor.

If you want to read a book that is close to the truth and will fill you with righteous indignation I recommend Grisham's "The appeal". His subject matter is so closely linked to this book that I checked in the acknowledgement section but Dr. Davis' name doesn't appear. Could Grisham be accused of plagiarism or is this another episode of synchronicity in my life?

Breast Cancer

Chapter 26

Breast Cancer: A Personal Prologue

(World Breast Cancer Report 2012; Ed. Peter Boyle)

The first time I guessed that something was wrong with my mother was when I noticed her clasping her lower back in pain whilst climbing upstairs in front of me. This was in about 1972 on one of my rare visits home during my period of living in Cardiff and the image is burnt in my memory as a result of what was to follow. My mother was extremely stoical and never complained about ill health. Following on my enquiry, she claimed that it was her "rheumatism" playing up. I thought no more about it until about three months later when she was admitted to hospital to have her gall bladder removed because of stones and increasing pains in the region just below the ribs on the right. This was in no way alarming or for that matter surprising, as she fitted the stereotype. She was female, overweight and over forty. In addition she was constantly munching "Rennies" for heartburn, presumably due to reflux oesophagitis, which tends to co-exist with gallstones. The operation went all right and she did indeed have gall stones; however in the post operative phase she developed agonizing pain spreading round from her mid lumbar region to the upper abdomen. X rays of her spine showed a crush fracture of the first lumbar vertebra and suspicion of skeletal secondaries from an unsuspected cancer. A rapid and more thorough clinical examination revealed an advanced cancer in her right breast. She was told not to worry as this was only "chronic mastitis" but my father was contacted immediately and told the grim news. My dad then contacted his five children, three of whom were medically qualified, to pass on the news, and begged us not to let on to mum that she had cancer that had spread round the body. To my lasting shame I concurred with this charade. Opiates were the only way of controlling her pain in the short term although radiotherapy to the spine provided more lasting benefit. The chemotherapy was harsh, causing nausea, vomiting, fatigue and the permanent loss of her long glossy black hair. I was not aware of any benefit from this cruel cocktail. After about twelve months the pains started up again and became more and more difficult to control. It reached the point when, according to erroneous belief at the time, that adequate analgesia would suppress her breathing and accelerate her demise, escalating doses of opiates were denied her. She therefore continued to suffer until neither she nor the family could take any more and she died within 6 hours of a dose of morphine that adequately controlled her pain. She died on my 37th birthday, May 31st 1974.

The Jewish tradition has it that the dead must be buried within 24 hours and until then the body must not be left alone. I spent the nightlong vigil with my father and had plenty of time to confront my conscience, firstly for not having done enough to help her and secondly for not having demonstrated a son's love at the time she needed it most.

Every mother loves her sons unconditionally but the return of such love by a son is often conditional and context dependent. At the time of my mother's terminal illness I was very self absorbed. My duties as a senior lecturer/consultant surgeon at the University Hospital of Wales were onerous and occupied me for about ten hours a day not counting a one in three rota for night time emergencies. I was very ambitious, setting up research programs; raising grants and keeping my eyes open for the chance of a professorial appointment. I often worked all weekends keeping up to date with the medical journals, writing manuscripts and dealing with correspondence. What little time I had left was lavished on my wife and three children under 7. I had no more space for love beyond this narrow circle and resented the distraction of my mother's illness at the time. I loved her as a dependent child, was embarrassed by her hats on parent's day when I was a school boy, had little time for her as a young professional but came to admire and yes, love her most of all, in retrospect, since her death.

My mother was a true *ayshet chayil* (a woman of worth) who dedicated her whole life to the family, the most selfless person I have ever known. During the dark days of the war, the blitz and rationing, she looked after four children of her own (my sister was born after the war) together with other orphans, waifs and strays. From negligible resources she conjured up spectacular *haimishe* (homely) meals, made her own cream cheese, *lokshen* (noodles) and *kichelers* (biscuits) from basic raw materials. In the absence of any household appliances she boiled all the linen in a great bubbling cauldron of a tub, extracted the last mote of dirt from the wet clothing and bed sheets on a scrubbing board, squeezed out the water in a huge mangle like a primitive printing press and hung it all out to dry either in the roof on a pulley system or if the weather was fine on a line in the yard. The heavy pre-modern irons were heated on the hot surface of the range (a pre-modern kind of Aga) and heaved on to the ironing board that was in constant use. Her obsessive personality (something I've inherited with a vengeance) meant that everything had to be folded and filed away in its place before she collapsed into bed after midnight. By the time I rose in the morning, the coke-fuelled range was alight, water had been boiled and a hearty breakfast prepared to keep us insulated from the cold on our walk to school.

She was not a conventionally beautiful woman, but apple cheeks, dimples and an endearing smile, radiated warmth and internal loveliness. From her forties onwards she was stout, but in those days even the most fashion conscious women relied on whalebone rather than "weightwatchers" to define their waist and redistribute the fat above and below the belt. She was always smartly "turned out" and would never be seen out of doors without makeup and a feather in her rakish hat. Most of all though she prided herself on her long black hair, which she assured me, came down to her waist. I could never confirm this, as she was too proud to leave her bedroom without her hair fixed up in a complex chignon secured in place like a Japanese Geisha girl. The loss of her hair and its replacement with a silk scarf, was the final insult that the cancer could hurl at her and for what purpose?

One evening 20 years after my mother's death, I received a phone call from my sister Linda, and then aged 48. She explained that she had just noticed a lump in her right breast, her GP had referred her to the local surgeon who had reassured her but arranged for a biopsy in about two months time. By this time I was Professor of surgery at the Royal Marsden Hospital in London, the most prestigious specialist cancer centre in the UK. I swallowed hard and suggested that she got a second opinion from Mr. Nigel Sacks, a man I trusted because as my senior lecturer I had witnessed the care and skill of his practice first hand. It has to be understood that I couldn't examine my own sister or trust my own judgment, in part out of decorum and in part out of emotional involvement. He saw her the next day and completed the "triple assessment";

that is clinical examination, X rays and a needle biopsy. Within the hour her cancer was diagnosed! Within the week she had surgery that consisted of a "lumpectomy" and partial excision of the lymph nodes in her right axilla. She was home in two days and happily the pathology was favorable. The margins of excision were clear of disease, the tumour was low grade and hormone receptor positive and finally the lymph nodes were declared free of malignant deposits. She was started on tamoxifen which she took without side effects for 5 years and underwent a 6 weeks course of radiotherapy to the breast. Without tempting providence I'm happy to say that 18 years later she is still alive and well and still my lovely sister Linda, who follows in my mother's footsteps as an *ayshet chayil.* She has four vivacious daughters who I adore and I think they reciprocate my love.

Without wishing to over-dramatize the case, I feel that to some extent I've expunged a little of the guilt I felt over my failure to help my mother. I transferred my sister's care to a top specialist and expedited her diagnosis and treatment. Most of all I have to take some satisfaction in having lead the team that first demonstrated that the drug, tamoxifen could reduce breast cancer mortality.

I now have to worry about the next two generations. I have two daughters and one granddaughter. My oldest brother has one daughter and three granddaughters. My second oldest brother has two daughters and two granddaughters whilst my sister has four daughters and two granddaughters: that's 17 young women living at an increased risk of the disease!

A few years ago Linda's oldest daughter, came to see me for advice. I'm sure she wouldn't mind me describing her as theatrical in all senses of the word, but on this occasion I felt that her anxieties were legitimate. Her mother and grandmother had breast cancer and the circumstances of her great grandmother's death also gave rise to concern. In addition we are of *Ashkenazi* extraction. All this hinted at the possibility of a germ line mutation in the BRCA gene pool which if present could lead to an 80% lifetime chance of developing breast cancer. I referred her on to my friend Ros Eeles, a leading cancer geneticist at the Royal Marsden Hospital, who agreed that the family pedigree did suggest a risk of carrying a breast cancer predisposition gene. With counseling and agreement from the whole family my sister was tested for the *"Ashkenazi"* mutations on BRCA 1 and BRCA 2. To everyone's relief Linda was not found to be a carrier.

This story of three generations of my family neatly encapsulates the evolving story of progress in the fight against breast cancer over the forty years since I got involved in the campaign.

My mother was too ignorant and or modest to be aware of the disease. Cancer the “big C” was not talked about or considered almost a stigma close to that associated with “a spot on the lung”, the euphemism for tuberculosis. Euphemisms for breast cancer were legion including chronic mastitis, neoplasia, mitotic lesions and at worst a “tumor”, that literally means nothing more than a swelling.

As a result of all this most cancers presented in a late stage either inoperable or with overt distant spread. Even if operable the surgery would be a mutilating Halsted radical mastectomy. With no malice intended, women where considered too emotionally labile to handle the truth, so the diagnosis and treatment were discussed with the husband and sons. (I used to encounter this cultural mind set with some of my private patients from Pakistan, Saudi Arabia and the Gulf states).

Finally palliative care and symptom control were poorly developed and patients suffered unnecessarily. The myth that adequate opiate analgesia shortens life has now been exploded; in fact the opposite is true. Too little and too late has been replaced by adequate and in good time.

By the time my sister presented breast cancer the subject was no longer stigmatized and breast cancer awareness campaigns were making their mark. Diagnosis was available in a “one stop shop” within the hour, matching “Quikfit” car exhaust replacement for efficiency.

Surgery in most cases can now provide breast conservation with a decent cosmetic outcome without compromising the chance of cure and adjuvant systemic therapy can prolong life or even provide a cure. The development of clinical nurse specialists and the subject of psychosocial-oncology have enhanced quality of life and the developments in palliative care and the hospice movement has improved quality of dying.

The experience with my niece provides a pointer to the future. The genetic code for the rare familial predisposition to breast cancer has been cracked. The mechanism that explains why a faulty gene can lead to cancer is understood and opportunities for prevention are opening up. Within a few years I expect the genetic explanation for sporadic breast cancers will be understood and along with that smart ways of preventing the disease will be discovered. In the immediate future we can expect more effective systemic therapy tailored to the individual cancer with specific molecular targets in its aim.

I now wish to take my families’ experience of breast cancer as a backdrop against which to judge my own professional development and the remarkable advances I’ve witnessed in the management of the disease.

It is of course difficult for me to be dispassionate because of my emotional involvement and also because like all clinical scientists I carry certain prejudices not shared by other equally wise men and women. I will describe this 40-year journey of discovery in the following sections of this book.

Chapter 27

The Natural History of Breast Cancer

(Breast Beating: A personal Odyssey in the quest for an understanding of breast cancer, the meaning of life and other easy questions. Anshan publishers Tunbridge Wells 2010)

Introduction

The expression "Natural History" has two meanings. Historically it has come to mean the systematic study of all natural objects, hence the famous collection of dinosaur skeletons, trilobite fossils and Darwin's specimens from the Galapagos Islands in the Natural History Museum, South Kensington, London.

Another meaning to this expression used as a medical term, is the behaviour of a disease in the absence of treatment or in other words *left to nature.*

In the modern world we accept the concept that many minor ailments are self limiting and jokingly reassure our friends that their bad cold will get better in a week, but with whiskey, a warm bed and tender loving care it will only take seven days. With more serious conditions that are life threatening or could lead to chronic dysfunction, we treat in order to influence this natural history in a favourable direction and rely on the history books to tell us what would have happened in the absence of treatment but with careful observation alone. Unfortunately in the days before active treatment of serious disease, careful and systematic observation, were also exceptional. And this applies in particular to carcinoma of the breast.

Another relevant issue here is that we don't always see in a dispassionate way the objective reality of that which we observe but more likely a distortion, refracted through the prism of our personal prejudices. Observations that reinforce our prejudices are embraced and those that challenge our beliefs are ignored or rationalized away.

But why should we have a prior set of beliefs so powerful as to impair our observation of something so fundamental as the natural history of a life threatening disease? The simple answer to that is "human nature".

Part of our success in evolution from the lower primates is the capacity to make order out of the myriad daily observations of our busy lives. We constantly but sub-consciously create hypotheses or models of objective reality- some are silly, most have a survival advantage and some in the fullness of time are found to have misled us all along.

However in this essay I wish to concentrate on the natural history of breast cancer and the evolution of conceptual models to explain its behaviour. I propose that all this is fundamental to improving the lot of our suffering patients for the simple reason that our treatments are the therapeutic consequence of our belief in the underlying mechanisms of disease. In other words belief systems and treatment modalities are two sides of the same coin.

The Nature of Models and Models of Nature

A model car we understand but a model of nature, what can that mean? Let me explain. Models are not just mechanical miniatures of the real thing; they can be anything else which helps to capture the very essence of the subject of our scrutiny. They can be metaphysical, mechanistic or mathematical; you can also include biological models of organic objects for good measure.

Let me illustrate this with two objects, one inorganic and the other organic.

Let us take that motor- car we cherish so much. Many sports car enthusiasts keep perfect replicas scaled down to 1:1,000 on their desks in preference to photographs of their wives and children. This is a mechanical model. Their wives view the contraption as the work of the devil; that if you like is a metaphysical model. Finally, the mechanical engineer can reproduce the energy of the internal combustion unit and the torque of the transmission system as mathematical formulae. That is a mathematical model.

My organic example is the rose bush I see from my study window and in particular one rose of an enchanting hue like the blush on the cheeks of Raphael's Madonna.

"What's in a name? That which we call a rose by any other name would smell as sweet", is a Shakespearian metaphysical model of this organic object.

Easier to handle is the mechanistic model in a children's primary school botany books. Here the rose is built up of petals, sepals, stamens, filament, anther and carpel all connected to a stalk with leaves, thorns and roots. It loses its poetry when broken down this way. Even more so when the reductionists do their worst and the rose is described as a molecular model. Curiously enough much of the beauty and mystery of the rose reappears in its mathematical model.

The new mathematics of Fibonacci numbers, fractals and Lindenmayer systems allow us to generate beautiful floribunda on our computer screens thus linking the mathematical model of the rose to the greater symmetries and complex patterns of all of God's creation. [1]

The Natural History of an Automobile and a Rose

Left to nature an automobile will rust and its engine will seize up. As our knowledge of the automobile and of the mechanism of rusting developed in tandem we have a ready explanation for this process, which is well understood.

The chemical reaction between iron and oxygen in the presence of moisture leads to corrosion and the production of iron oxide (Fe2O3). We can influence this natural history by keeping the car dry, well oiled and locked away. With luck the automobile will now last us up to 20 years: its maximum expectation of life.

The rose has a different and much more complex natural history. Left to nature it will enjoy an annual cycle of renewal, flowering every summer, resting every winter and springing into bud each spring. In addition left to nature, it grows into angry knots; it develops suckers with seven leaves instead of five on each stem, which grow to prodigious lengths. Then holes appear in the leaves, brown patches of rust add to their disfigurement and greenflies infest and destroy the buds. In the bad old days you could accuse your neighbour of witchcraft for blighting your bushes (a metaphysical model of disease) but in this modern era I know that the "rust" is a fungus (*Puccinia basdiomycetes)* and the holes are thanks to the caterpillars. I can influence this natural history with the aid of scientific horticulture, by pruning in February, putting phosphates down in March and spraying with inorganic chemicals all summer. This way their expectation of life can be 40 to 50 years with blooms as big as cabbages.

Breast Cancer

After that long preamble, the relevance of which will become immediately clear, I wish to return to the natural history of breast cancer. If left untreated what would happen and of equal importance, why?

To start with I wish to describe two anecdotal case histories, one from the 17th century and one from the 21st.

In the Louvre, Paris hangs a large and beguiling masterpiece by Rembrant, "Bathsheba at her toilet". Completed in 1655, the painting shows a naked Bathsheba looking wistfully into the middle distance left, whilst holding a letter in her right hand. Her attendant bathes her feet in a pool and the background is dark and ambiguous. Perhaps she has just learnt of her husband's death in battle as a result of King's David's treachery, leaving her free to join the long list of the royal concubines. About 25 years ago whilst working as a senior lecturer in the department of surgery at the Welsh National School of Medicine in Cardiff, a young Australian research fellow, Peter Braithwaite, drew my attention to the dimple in the upper outer quadrant of Bathsheba's left breast. I had to agree with him that the model for this painting has the classical stigma of breast cancer, which I have confirmed on subsequent visits to the Louvre, to see the painting in the flesh, so to speak. I encouraged him to research the history of the painting and its model. His work on this ultimately appeared in print [2], since when Bathsheba has become an icon of the breast cancer movement. In short the model was Hendrejke Stoffles who doubled up as mistress and housekeeper for Rembrandt. She was in her thirties when the picture was completed and died eight years later. Her mode of dying was characteristic of breast cancer with secondaries to the liver. There is no record of her being treated, but in any case treatment in those days was a futile hocus -pocus based on the metaphysical doctrines of Aristotle and Galen, yet she lived eight years after the clinically obvious disease became apparent, unknowingly portrayed in the painting.

The second anecdote concerns a woman booked into my clinic at the Portland hospital a few months ago. She claimed to be an "old patient" yet my secretary had no record of her. It transpired that I had seen her on only one occasion and that was eight years previously at The Royal Marsden Hospital. Piecing the story together I suddenly recalled the visit. She was 49 at the time but was now 57. I had diagnosed multi-focal carcinoma of the left breast at biopsy and recommended a mastectomy to be followed by 5 years of tamoxifen. She firmly but politely declined my advice and, in her own words, placed herself in the hands of Jesus and the prayers of her evangelical community. Not believing in the power of prayer to heal, I confessed to surprise at seeing her alive and wanted to know how I could help. The only complaint to which she confessed was swelling of the left arm. Exchanging glances with her attentive husband and daughter I asked her to disrobe in the examination room bracing myself for the worst. Well it wasn't the worst I've seen but pretty gruesome nonetheless. Hard nodules of cancer now replaced both breasts and both axillae were full of the disease causing massive lymphoedema of the arms, yet there was no evidence of distant metastases. Not wishing to push my luck too far by asking for another biopsy I made the assumption that the tumour was hormone responsive and advised to start on anastrozole (Arimidex) suggesting that Jesus now needed a little help from modern medicine as prayer alone would no longer hold the cancer in check.

She politely took my prescription and promised to return in one month to check on progress. Needless to say she failed to keep that appointment.

Of course at the other extreme I have witnessed many women who presented "early" were treated promptly yet died within two years.

Breast Cancer in the 19thC and Early 20thC

In 1970 whilst working with Dr Bernard Fisher in Pittsburgh, I visited the library of the NIH in Bethesda with the object of completing an historical review for my thesis. Whilst searching for one reference a more important one literally fell in my lap. This happened to be a treatise on breast cancer by Dr. Gross of Philadelphia published in 1880 [3]. Gross' treatise provides a clear insight into the status of the disease in the era immediately before the developments in anaesthesia and antisepsis which allowed surgeons to attempt a radical cure of breast cancer. He describes a series of 616 cases, 70% of whom had skin infiltration on presentation which had ulcerated through in 25% of the patients. 64% had extensive involvement of axillary nodes and

27% had obvious supra-clavicular nodal involvement. Accepting that the meagre benefits of surgery seldom outweighed the risks in those days, he judged it ethical to follow the natural course of 97 cases who received nothing other than “constitutional support”.

He describes how skin infiltration appeared on average 14 months after a tumour is first detected, ulceration appears on average six months after that, fixation to the chest wall after a further two months and invasion of the other breast if the patient lived on average 32 months after the lump first appeared. The average time for the appearance of enlarged axillary nodes was 15 months in those few cases that presented with an “empty” axilla to start with. 25% of all these untreated cases exhibited obvious distant metastases within a year and 25% after three years with only 5% surviving more than 5 years.

Since then a number of different series of untreated breast cancer have been reported. For example, Greenwood in 1226 [4] described a 6 year follow up of 651 cases of untreated breast cancer with only 60 remaining alive at the end of this period. Daland in 1927[5] reported a series of 100 patients who were considered inoperable, unfit for surgery or who had refused the offer of surgery. The average duration of life was 40 months for the whole group, 43 months for those deemed operable at diagnosis and 29 months for those deemed inoperable.

The study that has attracted the most attention over the years was that of Julian Bloom published in 1968 [6]. His data came from the records of 250 women dying of breast cancer in the Middlesex Hospital Cancer ward between 1905 and 1933. Of this group 95% died of breast cancer, but it should be noted that almost all of them presented with locally advanced or overt metastatic disease. The survival rates from the *alleged* onset of symptoms were 18% at 5 years, 0.8% at 15 years, with a mean survival of about two and a half years. The reason for withholding treatment are also worthy of note: old age or infirmity 35%; disease too advanced 30%; treatment refused 20%; and early death the remainder.

Although of historical interest I can’t really believe that these studies help to provide a baseline against which to judge the curative effect of modern treatment. Firstly, as with all retrospective uncontrolled series there has to be an element of selection. Why was treatment withheld? It is quite obvious that in the majority of these cases, with the exception of those refusing treatment, they all had an exceptionally poor prognosis to begin with. Secondly, they mostly represent women seeking medical attention at a time in the late 19thC or early 20thC, when many women were content to co-exist with their lump in blissful ignorance until they died of old age or were knocked down by a Hansom cab!

Next, the accuracy of the diagnosis might be called into question in the days before modern microscopy and the widespread adoption of the histological criteria of cancer.

Finally, for all we know the biological nature of the disease might have changed over the last 50 years as the incidence has increased following the major upheavals of demographic change and the widespread adoption of the oral contraceptive pill and HRT. [7]

It would of course be inconceivable to suggest we study an untreated group today and the closest approximation we can find comes from a report of the Ontario cancer clinics between 1938 and 1956, just preceding the jump in breast cancer incidence in the developed world. [8] Close on 10,000 cases were analyzed accounting for 40% of all new cases arising in the province of Ontario during this period. Amongst this group were 145 well -documented cases who received no treatment of any kind. Although, yet again 100 of these cases were untreated because of late stage of presentation or poor general condition, the rest were unable or unwilling to attend for treatment. A careful note was made of the date the patient first became aware of the lump from which point survival rates were computed. The 5year survival from first recorded symptom was 35% with a median survival of 47 months. The most surprising figure was a near 70% 5 year survival for the small group presenting with localized disease!

This then raises the inevitable question, is carcinoma of the breast inevitably a fatal disease if neglected? This question is almost impossible to answer with confidence although hinted at by anecdotal evidence. In addition to the case described above I have experience of four other well- documented cases refusing treatment for 7,10,13 and 16 years respectively. One eventually died of stomach cancer with a still localized cancer within the breast weighing an estimated 2 Kg. However, the best documented in the literature was reported by Steckler and Martin in 1973 [9].

They described a 38-year-old woman with histologically proven cancer who refused surgery and was then followed up for 20 years before consenting. We will never know how many of the cases we see in our daily practice carry such a favorable natural history.

The Influence of Surgery on the Natural History of Breast Cancer

From the popularization of the classical radical mastectomy at the very end of the 19thC [10] until about 1975 almost all patients with breast cancer of a technically operable stage were treated with modifications of the radical mastectomy. To those without commitment to a prior hypothesis, this allowed for new insights about the nature of the malignant process. Before considering this matter it's worth revisiting the conceptual model that allowed the radical operation to reign supreme for 75 years.

Until the discovery of the microscope and the eventual correlation between cancer and its microscopic appearance (c late 18th early 19thC), breast cancer was ascribed to an imbalance of the metaphysical "natural humours" first proposed by Aristotle in 5thC BC Athens and then elaborated upon by Galen in the Greco- Roman period of the 2ndC AD. [11] It was asserted that the disease was an accumulation of black bile, "melancholia", in the breast. Support for this view was the fact that women with breast cancer were "melancholic" (one must question the direction of causality here) and that the disease increased in frequency after the cessation of the menses which allowed "black bile" to accumulate. The therapeutic consequences of this belief involved bizarre diets, cupping, venesection and purgation with exotic enemas (some of these excesses are still practiced by the lunatic fringe of the alternative brigade). Failures were dismissed as loss of nerve by the patient or physician; if death followed over zealous bleeding this showed lack of gratitude by the patient who at least died free of melancholia!

In about 1840, Virchow described a revolutionary model of the disease, building on the development of microscopy and post-mortem examinations of the cadavers of breast cancer victims. [12] He suggested that the disease started as a single focus within the breast, expanding with time and then migrating along lymphatic channels to the lymph glands in the axilla. These glands were said to act as a first line of defence filtering out the cancer cells. Once these filters became saturated the glands themselves acted as a nidus for tertiary spread to a second and then third line of defence like the curtain walls around a medieval citadel. Ultimately when all defences were exhausted the disease spread along tissue planes to the skeleton and vital organs.

The therapeutic consequences of this belief had to await the development of anaesthesia and antisepsis in the 1880s but were seized upon by Halsted in about 1895 with his complete experience being described in 1932. [13] Armed with these insights, it seemed inevitable that patients would be cured by radical operations that cut away all of the breast, the overlying skin, the underlying muscles and as many lymph node groups compatible with survival. So convincing were these arguments and so charismatic their chief proponent, the Halsted operation was adopted as default therapy all round the world. At this long perspective we are entitled to ask to what extent did the radical operation add to the curability of the disease and what can we learn about the nature of the beast by its behaviour following such mutilating surgery? We can also add a third question concerning human nature and our unwillingness to see facts "which almost slap us in the face" * [14] William Halsted operated at a time when the triumph of mechanistic principles was at its peak. The common man had begun enjoying the fruits of the Industrial Revolution. Naturally, Halsted's 'complete operation' was based on straightforward concepts about the behaviour of cancer, more mechanistic than biological.

("It is now, as it was then, as it may ever be, conceptions from the past blind us to facts which almost slap us in the face"* - WS Halsted 1908)

His surgical expertise was remarkable, and for the first time, breast cancer seemed curable with recurrence rates (6% local + 14% regional) at 3 years of follow-up, very low compared to the other series at that time.

Halsted's pioneering work in breast cancer served as a model for many other solid cancers and his principles are still successful in cancers such as squamous cell carcinomas of the head and neck, "the commando operation", and cervix, "Wertheim's operation". Unfortunately, only 23% of patients treated by Halsted survived 10 years [13]. The natural response to this failure was even more radical surgery. Internal mammary lymph nodes that received about 25% of the lymphatic drainage of the breast were not removed in the 'complete operation' but included in the super radical operations that followed, or in the fields of radiation after surgery.

Retrospective studies indicated that more radical operations improved survival [15]. However, in randomized trials that followed later, no benefit could be demonstrated [16,17]. Thus even when the tumor seemed to have been completely 'removed with its roots', the patients still developed distant metastases and succumbed: 30% of node negative and 75% of node-positive patients eventually dying of the disease over 10 years when they were treated by radical surgery alone [18] and with no evidence of "cure" if patients were followed up for 25 years. [19] In this latter seminal study by Brinkley and Haybittle, a group of over 700 breast cancer patients, treated by radical surgery alone and followed up for 25 years, continued to demonstrate an excess mortality compared to an aged matched population.

The Biological Revolution of the Late 20thC

Prompted by the failures of radical operations to cure patients of breast cancer, Fisher proposed a revolutionary hypothesis that rejected the mechanistic models of the past. [20] He postulated that cancer spreads via the blood stream even before its clinical detection, with the outcome determined by the biology of tumor–host interactions. Based on this concept of 'biological predeterminism', he predicted the following: (A) The extent of local treatment would not affect survival; and (B) systemic treatment of even seemingly localized tumours would be beneficial and might even offer a chance of cure.

Several pioneers in the field set up randomized clinical trials to test these hypotheses culminating in a series of world overviews. [21] Although the "Fisherian" doctrine is now taken as 'proven', we must accept that the proof is more in principle rather than in cure. The benefits from systemic therapy are modest, with a relative risk reduction in breast cancer mortality of about 25% overall, which translates to about 8–10% in absolute terms. As regards the extent of local treatment, many randomized trials have tested less versus more surgery with or without adjuvant radiotherapy.

A recent world overview of these trials [22] concluded that more radical local treatment; surgery or adjuvant radiotherapy does not have any influence on the appearance of distant disease and overall survival with one caveat (*vide infra)*. This is in spite of the increase in local recurrence rates with less radical local treatment, i.e. although radical surgery or postoperative radiotherapy had a substantial effect on reducing local recurrence rates, it did not improve overall or distant disease-free survival.

All the above can be taken as powerful corroboration of Fisher's theory that metastases of any importance have already occurred *before* the clinical or radiological detection in about 90% of all breast cancers.

Phenomena That Challenge the Existing Models

Local Treatment

Even in the world overview there is one finding that was not completely in keeping with Fisher's doctrine of biological predeterminism. Radiotherapy does actually reduce the breast cancer-specific deaths by about 3%—only to be counterbalanced by the increased mortality from late cardiac complications in those patients with cancer in the left breast because of radiation damage to the heart.

More recently, two randomized-controlled trials evaluated the value of postoperative radiotherapy after mastectomy for tumors with a poor prognosis. The radiotherapy techniques in these two studies minimized the dose to the heart. Not surprisingly, there was a reduction in local recurrence rates, but there was also an improvement in the overall 10-year survival rates—9% [25] and 10% [26]. The most likely explanation for this large difference in survival rates could be a statistical quirk.

Let us assume that radiotherapy does impart a small survival benefit. When several trials are conducted, the different magnitudes of effects seen are expected to follow a normal distribution. A sufficiently large trial would be highly likely to detect this small difference, whereas a small trial will rarely yield a positive result because of type II error. The effect in a small trial will need to be larger than the real effect (just by chance) for it to be detected at all, consequently small trials that are positive will usually be those which reveal a larger than real effect.

Whatever the explanations for the magnitude of effect in these trials, it is clear that more extensive local treatment is not completely ineffective in improving survival. This could mean that local recurrence ***is*** a source of tertiary spread, although the metastases arising from the primary tumour at the point of diagnosis exert most of the prognostic influence. Or alternatively, it is merely a marker of a radio-resistant tumour with a poor prognosis: the local recurrence being an expression rather than a determinant of distant relapse.

Adjuvant Systemic Therapy Has Only a Modest Effect on Survival

The development of adjuvant systemic therapeutic regimens was based on the kinetics of tumour growth and its response to chemotherapy in animal models [27]. However, the early clinical trials predicted a large benefit and were consequently underpowered to detect the modest 'real' benefit. Consequently, there was considerable confusion, with the positive results of some of the early trials being contradicted by negative or equivocal results of others. The overview analysis, however, confirmed that adjuvant systemic therapy can in fact be beneficial [21]. It is the magnitude of benefit that is disappointingly modest—an absolute benefit of a maximum of 12% in high-risk premenopausal individuals and of 2% in equivalent-risk postmenopausal individuals is much smaller than anticipated from the experimental models.

The next step taken by medical oncologists was very similar in attitude to that taken by surgeons only a few decades ago, if a little doesn't work then try a lot!

This approach was bolstered by the excellent rate of long-term cure achieved in haematological malignancies. In addition, tumour cell lines showed a log-linear dose response when exposed to alkylating agents [28,29].

Needless to say the high dose chemotherapy with bone marrow rescue was a failure and the least said about this sorry episode in the history of breast cancer the better, yet there maybe lessons to learn from the failure of this approach.

When Does a Primary Tumor Seed Its Secondaries?

If we believe that once a primary tumor gains access to the vasculature it starts seeding metastases in a linear or exponential manner, it should be expected that because a larger tumor has been in the body for a longer time, and therefore has had access to the vasculature for longer than smaller tumors, a much higher percentage of patients with larger tumors should present with metastases. This is true to some extent with regard to lymphatic metastases, i.e. there is a correlation of number of involved lymph nodes with the size of the primary tumour. However, this relationship is far from linear. Thus there are small or even occult tumours that have several involved lymph nodes, while many large tumours are found not to have metastasized to the axilla. This discrepancy becomes even more apparent when we consider distant metastases. It would be expected that the proportion of patients presenting with distant metastases would be higher for those with larger tumours as opposed to those with smaller tumours. Nevertheless, in real life a patient presenting with a primary tumour along with distant metastases is uncommon, however large the tumour. In fact, the percentages of patients that present with symptomatic metastases is 0%, 3% and 7% in stages I, II and III of the primary tumour, respectively [30]. However, when you look at the incidence of metastases in these same groups 18 months after their primary diagnosis and therapy, there is a clear correlation of primary tumour size with the proportion of patients experiencing distant relapse.

How can this be explained without challenging the linear model of breast cancer spread?

One explanation would be that although the number of metastases that are seeded by the primary tumour would be linearly related to the tumour size and biological aggressiveness, the *clinical* appearance of metastases is triggered *only* after the primary tumour has been disturbed or removed.

A modern theory that better explains tumour dormancy, would suggest that the micrometastases can remain *latent* for long periods of time, with a potential to grow *or regress,* in response to some systemic trigger.

Judah Folkman [31] has demonstrated that the critical balance of factors stimulating and inhibiting angiogenesis are very important in maintaining the balance between proliferation and apoptosis. When this balance is disturbed, the metastases can either grow, or completely disappear according to whether the *microenvironment* favours proliferation or programmed cell death. One likely trigger for 'kick-starting' the growth of micro-metastases, could be the act of surgery itself. After all in evolutionary terms an angiogenic response to trauma must facilitate healing in all sites of the body. Furthermore many tumours secrete anti-angiogenic factors that circulate in the body and inhibit angiogenesis in these latent metastases: an almost sinister evolutionary concept favouring the cancer—as if the primary tumour suppresses the outgrowth of micrometastases to keep its host alive!

Another way to examine this phenomenon is to consider the timing of recurrence and metastasis after primary therapy. This reveals a striking pattern that is usually expressed in terms of 'hazards'. Hazards are calculated by dividing the number of events in a particular time frame, say 6 months, by the number of patients at risk of having those events at the start of the period. In all clinical trials it is found that the hazards for metastasis and death rise sharply at 2–3 years after the primary diagnosis and then fall rising to a second peak at about 7–9 years [32]. It is extraordinary that this is true for any stage of the disease. The first peak occurs at the same time, whether the tumour was at stage I or stage III on diagnosis. It is only the amplitude of the peak that changes with stage, the later the stage the higher is the peak, but the timing of the signal remains the same.

These phenomena suggest a nonlinear dynamic model for breast cancer, which, like a chaotic system, is exquisitely sensitive to events around the time of diagnosis. It might even suggest that surgery could be responsible for accelerating the clinical appearance of metastatic disease. However, a randomized trial of surgery versus no surgery to prove this would no doubt be judged unethical in the absence of systemic therapy. Nevertheless, such a model is fortuitously available in the setting of randomized trials of mammographic screening [23].

A New Model to Explain the Natural History of Breast Cancer

Taking all this into account I would like to develop a new model to explain the natural history of the disease which in addition to explaining the success of the Fisherian model of "biological predeterminism" also explains the clinical observations that fail to fit neatly into the contemporary paradigm.

First of all, cancer should be seen as a process, not a morphological entity. [33] Individual cancers, while likely to originate from single cells, are constantly adapting to the local environment. There is no single substance or metabolic defect that is unique to cancer. Clonality, previously considered a hallmark of cancer, is neither always demonstrated in malignancy nor restricted to it [34]. The cancer cell is largely normal, both genetically and functionally.

The malignant properties are the result of a small number of genetic and/or environmental changes that have a profound effect on certain aspects of its behaviour. The three main processes of cancer, growth, invasion and metastasis, have their equivalents in normal tissues. Most cancers are diagnosed by virtue of their morphological or histochemical *similarity* to the tissue of origin. At the genetic level, with the exception of deletions, all necessary information is preserved, and the defective portion of DNA is small. The key processes of malignancy are genetically controlled by the under or over expression of normal genes and their products that normally serve essential cellular functions.

In addition, pathological and autopsy studies have suggested that most of the occult tumours in breast (and prostate cancers) may never reach clinical significance [35, 36].

Demicheli and colleagues [37] have also argued that a continuous growth model of breast cancer fails to explain the clinical data. The continuous growth model yielded tumour sizes too large to be missed at the preceding negative physical examinations, and required growth rates significantly lower than those consistent with clinical data. As mentioned before, the continuous growth model also fails to explain the biphasic recurrence pattern seen when hazards of recurrence are plotted for every year after diagnosis.

The new model is based on the concept of tumour dormancy/latency both in the preclinical phase within the breast and later with the micrometastases that seed in the early phase of the natural history of the disease, once the primary focus has developed it's microvasculature. The latter remain dormant until some signal; perhaps the act of surgery or other adverse life event stimulates them into fast growth.

Groups of cells without angiogenic potential can grow but remain small (up to 10^5 or 10^6cells). The metastatic focus may grow quickly if (i) a subset of these cell switches to an angiogenic phenotype and/or (ii) the inhibition of angiogenesis is removed. The model suggests that the metastatic development of unperturbed breast cancer is a sequential evolution from a non-angiogenic to an angiogenic state, with stochastic transitions from one state to the next.

This model may explain the early peak of hazard function for local and distant recurrences in resected cancer patients by combining with the *natural* metastatic development of unperturbed disease ("the Fisher effect") with the angiogenic signal following surgery ("the Folkman effect"). It also correlates well with the finding of a modest benefit after adjuvant systemic chemotherapy.

We can now add a new mathematical model to the biological model described above. [38] Breast cancer is like a complex organism existing in a state of dynamic equilibrium within the host, the equilibrium being very precarious and close to a chaotic boundary. Furthermore, the mathematics to describe the natural history of these "organisms" invokes nonlinear dynamics or chaos theory. This model is the first attempt to apply the new mathematics of complexity to make predictions about the factors influencing the natural history of breast cancer that might one day provide a therapeutic window.

Central to the understanding of this model is the pioneering work of Folkman on tumour angiogenesis [39]. As we know, solid tumours cannot grow beyond 10^6 cells or about 1–2 mm in diameter in the absence of a blood supply [40]. The initial prevascular phase of growth is followed by a vascular phase in which tumour-induced angiogenesis is the rate-limiting step for further growth and provides malignant cells direct access to the circulation [41].

In addition to the importance of the microvasculature, we can also visualize these microscopic foci as existing in a 'soup' of cytokines, endocrine polypeptides and steroids, with cells interacting with each other and with the surrounding stroma, interpreting competing signals directing the cancer cells in the direction of proliferation or apoptosis.

Such complexity cannot be modelled by linear dynamics, or even a full understanding of the complete catalogue of genetic mutations at the cellular level, because the critical events of multiple cell-to-cell interactions require a thorough understanding of epigenetic phenomena.

With my mathematically literate colleagues I have tried to model this complex system. [38] Our model, like other 'chaotic systems', produces beautiful fractal-like images that can be shown to be exquisitely sensitive to initial conditions (e.g. different concentrations or different gradients of the three biological variables). The three-dimensional vasculature of a tumor as simulated by these formulae is very similar to the vasculature of a breast tumor visualized using three-dimensional computerized tomography (CT) reconstruction. [42]

There is ample scope for the addition of further complexity to the model, by incorporating more variables.

The therapeutic consequences of the new models are almost self-evident.

The intervention that suggests itself would be anti-angiogenic, and the timing of the intervention would be preoperative, so that at the time of surgery the system is primed to protect against sudden flooding with angiogenic signals. Indeed, some of the success attributed to adjuvant tamoxifen or chemotherapy might be a result of their anti-angiogenic potential rather cytostatic/cytocidal effects [43].

Assuming we can protect the subject from the first peak of metastatic outgrowth, we will then have to monitor her with extreme vigilance. By the time the metastases are clinically apparent it is perhaps too late, therefore monitoring the patient with tumour markers and reintroducing an anti-angiogenic strategy at the first rise in tumour markers might prove successful. [44]

In the meantime, we can continue to add additional layers of complexity to the simulations of our mathematical model to help develop alternative strategies for biological interventions to maintain the disease in equilibrium until nature takes its cull in old age. Unlike the hamster lymphoma models of the past, the new model feeds on complexity and becomes closer and closer to simulating nature in all her awesome beauty.

References

[1] Ian Stewart, Life's other secret: the new mathematics of the living world. Allen Lane The Penguin Press, London, 1998.

[2] Braithwaite PA and Shugg D, Rembrandt's Bathsheba: the dark shadow of the left breast. *Annals of the Royal College of Surgeons*. 1983;65: 337-339.

[3] Gross SW, A practical treatise of tumours of the mammary gland. D. Appelton & Co New York, 1880.

[4] Greenwood M, A report on the natural duration of cancer: reports on public health and medical subjects, No. 33 H.M.S.O. London, 1926.
[5] Daland EM, Untreated Carcinoma of the Breast. *Surgery, Gynaecology and Obstetrics,* 1927; 44: 264-271.
[6] Bloom HJG, Survival of women with untreated breast cancer-Past and present. In, Prognostic Factors in breast Cancer, Eds. *APM Forrest and PB Kunkler*, E&S Livingston Ltd. Edinburgh, 1968.
[7] Quinn MJ, Martinez-Garcia C, Berrino F, EUROCARE working group, Variations in survival from breast cancer in Europe by age and country, 1978-89. *European J Cancer* 1998; 34:2204-11
[8] MacKay EN and Sellers AH, Breast cancer at the Ontario Cancer Clinics, 1938-56, A statistical review. Medical statistics branch, Ontario department of health. 1965.
[9] Steckler RM and Martin RG, Prolonged survival in untreated breast cancer. *The American J Surgery* 1973;126: 111-119.
[10] Halsted WS. The results of operations for the cure of cancer of the breast performed at The Johns Hopkins Hospital from June 1889 to January1894. *Johns Hopkins Hosp Rep* 1894; 4: 297–350.
[11] DeMoulin D, A short history of Cancer. Martinus Nyhoff Publishers, Boston, The Hague, Lancaster. 1983.
[12] Virchow R. 1863-1873 Die Krankhaften Geschwulste, Hirshwald Publishers, Berlin. Vol 1.
[13] Lewis D, Rienhoff WFJ. A study of results of operations for the cure of cancer of the breast. *Ann Surg* 1932;95: 336.
[14] Halsted WS The training of the Surgeon. In surgical papers by William Stewart Halsted, Vol. 2. The Johns Hopkins Press; Baltimore, 1924.
[15] Urban J. Management of operable breast cancer: the surgeon's view. *Cancer* 1978; 42: 2066.
[16] Meier P, Ferguson DJ, Karrison T. A controlled trial of extended radical mastectomy. *Cancer* 1985; 55: 880–91.
[17] Lacour J, Le M, Caceres E, Koszarowski T, Veronesi U, Hill C. Radical mastectomy versus radical mastectomy plus internal mammary dissection. Ten year results of an international cooperative trial in breast cancer. *Cancer* 1983; 51: 1941–3.
[18] Brinkley D and Haybittle JL. A 15 year follow up study of patients treated for carcinoma of the breast. *British J Radiology*, 1968;41:215-221 Brinkley D and Haybittle JL. The curability of breast cancer. *The Lancet* 1975;2:9-14.

[19] Fisher B. Laboratory and clinical research in breast cancer: a personal adventure: the David A. Karnofsky memorial lecture. *Cancer Res* 1980;40: 3863–74.
[20] Early Breast Cancer Trialists' Collaborative Group. Systemic treatment of early breast cancer by hormonal, cytotoxic or immune therapy: 133 randomized trials involving 31,000 recurrences and 24,000 deaths among 75,000 women. *Lancet* 1992;339:1-15,71-85.
[21] Early Breast Cancer Trialists' Collaborative Group. Effects of radiotherapy and surgery in early breast cancer. An overview of randomized trials. *N Engl J Med* 1995; 333:1444–5.
[22] Nystrom L, Andersson I, Bjurstam L, et al, Long term effects of mammographic screening: updated overview of the Swedish randomized trials. *Lancet*; 2002;359:909-919.
[23] Götzche PC, Olsen O, Is screening for breast cancer by mammography justifiable?. Lancet 2000; 355:129-34
[24] Overgaard M, Hansen PS, Overgaard J *et al.* Postoperative radiotherapy in high-risk premenopausal women with breast cancer who receive adjuvant chemotherapy. Danish Breast Cancer Cooperative Group 82b Trial *N Engl J Med* 1997;337: 949–55.
[25] Ragaz J, Jackson SM, Le N *et al* .Adjuvant radiotherapy and chemotherapy in node-positive premenopausal women with breast cancer. *N Engl J Med* 1997; 337: 956–62.
[26] Skipper HE. Kinetics of mammary tumor cell growth and implications for therapy. *Cancer* 1971; 28: 1479–99.
[27] Frei E III, Teicher B, Holden SA, Cathart KNS, Wang Y. Preclinical studies and clinical correlation of the effect of alkylating dose. *Cancer Res* 1988; 48: 6417–23.
[28] Frei E III, Antman K, Teicher B, Eder P, Schnipper L. Bone marrow autotransplantation for solid tumours—prospects. *J Clin Oncol* 1989; 7: 515–26.
[29] Coleman RE, Rubens RD, Fogelman I. Reappraisal of the baseline bone scan in breast cancer. *J Nucl Med* 1988; 29: 1045–9.
[30] Folkman J. Angiogenesis in cancer, vascular, rheumatoid and other disease. *Nat Med* 1995; 1: 27–31.
[31] Baum M, Badwe RA. Does surgery influence the natural history of breast cancer? In: Wise H, Johnson HJ, eds. *Breast Cancer: Controversies in Management.* Armonk, NY: Futura, 1994: 61–9.
[32] Schipper H, Turley EA, Baum M. A new biological framework for cancer research. *Lancet* 1996; 348: 1149–51.

[33] Schipper H. Historic milestones in cancer biology: a few that are important in cancer treatment. *Semin Oncol* 1979;6: 506–14.

[34] Baum M, Vaidya JS, Mittra I. Multicentricity and recurrence of breast cancer. *Lancet* 1997; 349: 208.

[35] Whitmore WFJ. The natural history of prostate cancer. *Cancer* 1973; 32: 1104–12.

[36] Demicheli R, Retsky MW, Swartzendruber DE, Bonadonna G. Proposal for a new model of breast cancer metastatic development. *Ann Oncol* 1997; 8: 1075–80.

[37] Baum M, Chaplain M, Anderson A, Douek M, Vaidya JS. Does breast cancer exist in a state of chaos? *Eur J Cancer* 1999; 35: 886–91.

[38] Folkman J. Tumor angiogenesis: therapeutic implications. *N Engl J Med* 1971; 285: 1182–6.

[39] Folkman J, Watson K, Ingber D, Hanahan D. Induction of angiogenesis during the transition from hyperplasia to neoplasia. *Nature* 1989; 339:58–61.

[40] Folkman J. What is the evidence that tumors are angiogenesis dependent? [editorial]. *J Natl Cancer Inst* 1990; 82: 4–6.

[41] Douek M, Davidson T, Hall-Craggs MA *et al.* Contrast enhancement MRI and tumour angiogenesis in breast cancer. *Br J Surg* 1997; 84: 1588.

[42] Haran E, Maretzek A, Goldberg I, Horowitz A, Degani H. Tamoxifen enhances cell death in implanted MCF7 breast cancer by inhibiting endothelial growth. *Cancer Res* 1994;54: 5511–14.

[43] Baum M, Benson JR Current and future roles of adjuvant endocrine therapy in management of early carcinoma of the breast. In Senn HJ, Gelber RD, Goldhirsch A, Thurlimann B, eds. *Recent Results in CancerResearch—Adjuvant Therapy of Breast Cancer.* Heidelberg: Springer, 1996:215–226.

Chapter 28

Breast Cancer Awareness as a Prerequisite for Reducing Mortality in Resource Poor Parts of the World

(Annals of Medicine and Surgery
Volume 1, Complete, Pages 16-18, 2012)

When I first started practicing as a surgeon it was commonplace to see women presenting with locally advanced or metastatic disease.

Unless young surgeons go and practice in sub-Saharan Africa or rural India, they are unlikely to witness the terrible ulcers and terrible smells of uncontrolled local disease. Fortunately over the last 30 years such sights are rare in our clinics. I think we can reasonably suggest that this is thanks to the work of the cancer charities promoting breast cancer awareness (BCA) in the resource rich parts of the world. BCA is not the same as "Breast self examination" (BSE). BSE is now discredited, as it is associated with an excess of unnecessary biopsies with no associated fall in mortality. [1] BCA is also in danger of overselling itself, as Breast Cancer Awareness month is transformed into "Black October", as more and more frightened young women overload our clinics because the women's magazines and the posters of the cancer charities carry pictures of nubile young women instead of examples of the women truly at risk e.g. overweight and of a certain age. That aside, programs of public health education in the poorest parts of the world would be cost effective in reducing morbidity and mortality of the disease. Screening is the very last thing such countries need, where most women present with stage III and IV of the disease. One step up from that being piloted in India by the WHO, is clinical breast examination (CBE) by field workers trained in simple techniques of clinical examination. [2] If only my mother had been breast cancer aware she might have lived to a ripe old age.

References

[1] Hackshaw, A. and E. Paul, Breast self-examination and death from breast cancer: a meta-analysis. *Br J Cancer*, 2003. 88: p. 1047-1053.

[2] Kösters JP, Gøtzsche PC. Regular self-examination or clinical examination for early detection of breast cancer. *Cochrane Database of Systematic Reviews* 2003, Issue 2. Art. No.: CD003373. DOI:10.1002 /14651858.CD003373

Chapter 29

Surgery for Breast Cancer: Shifting Paradigms and Scientific Revolutions

(World Breast Cancer Report 2012
European Inst for Prevention of Cancer)

The remarkable advances in the treatment of breast cancer I've witnessed over the last 40 years would never have come about without the conceptual revolution (paradigm shift) spearheaded by Dr. Bernard Fisher in Pittsburg in the late 1960s and early 1970s. The year I spent with him (1970/71) changed my whole approach to the epistemology of medicine in general and breast cancer in particular.

Up until the eighteenth century breast cancer was treated according to the principles of Galen with bloodletting, purgation and leeches. It wasn't until the mid-nineteenth century that it became widely accepted that cancer was a disease of cellular pathology originating within the breast and spreading centrifugally along the lymphatic system. The therapeutic consequence of this belief led surgeons to embark on radical surgery that involved removing the breast and all the regional lymphatics. It was left to William Halsted in the 1890s to refine the operation into the classic radical mastectomy, with the intention of ridding the body of the primary cancer and its lymph node secondaries. Sadly, the only support for this radical treatment was anecdotal. If the patient survived it was due to the success of the surgeon. If the patient died it was either because the patient came too late or the surgeon lacked the courage of his convictions to complete a truly radical operation. Between 1965 and 1970 I became adept at this mutilating procedure and prided myself that I could complete it without the need of a blood transfusion.

It was only when Dr Bernard Fisher in the late 1960s challenged the conceptual model of the disease that progress started to be made. In other words an antithesis was constructed to challenge the prevailing dogma. Fisher taught that contrary to popular belief, breast cancer cells spread throughout the body through the venous drainage of the breast, and at the time of clinical presentation of the disease, the majority of breast cancers were in fact systemic disorders. [1] If that was indeed the case then there were two therapeutic consequences. Firstly, that radical surgery is shutting the stable door after the horse has bolted. Therefore the role of local therapy is local control, which would equally well be achieved by breast conserving techniques such as lumpectomy and radiotherapy. The second therapeutic corollary is that if indeed the disease is systemic at the time of diagnosis then the only way to improve cure rates is through chemotherapy or hormone therapy. However, the greatness of Dr Fisher, ably supported by surgical acolytes all around the world, was not simply to accept a new set of beliefs in place of an old set of beliefs, but to challenge the new paradigm using deductive logic: in other words, through randomized controlled trials (RCTs). One of the great success stories of modern medicine has been the painstaking series of RCTs in the management of early breast cancer over the past 30 years. We now know with extreme confidence that breast conservation is a safe alternative to radical mastectomy, although not in itself improving cure rates, greatly enhancing the patient's quality of life. We also know with extreme confidence that treatment using either endocrine or cytotoxic regimens will improve survival. The final demonstration of that truth has been the dramatic fall in breast cancer mortality in the UK and North America since 1985, following the first publication of the world overview of trials. [2]

From Frozen Section to Triple Assessment

In the bad old days when I was taught to perform the classic radical mastectomy, the hors d'oeuvre before the surgical feast was the "frozen section". As an extension to the Halstedian doctrine, it was believed that manipulating or cutting into the tumor before its eradication would further express cancer cells into the afferent lymphatics. The poor victim would therefore have to sign consent, that if the lump in her breast turned out to be malignant on frozen section at the time of surgery, then the surgeon had permission to go ahead and take away her breast, pectoral muscles and lymph-nodes. This was even done for cases that were almost certainly fibroadenomata. Imagine the terror of the young woman waking up from the anaesthetic and checking to see if she still had two breasts. Apart from the insensitivity of this approach, it made it impossible for planning operating lists and organizing multi-disciplinary discussions before hand. Mind you in those days the surgeon was king, the radiotherapists his lackey and the medical oncologist had yet to be invented.

In many ways, both from the patient's and the clinician's perspective, one of the greatest advances I have witnessed has been the development of the triple assessment and the multi-disciplinary team (MDT) approach. Our specialist breast clinics are now organized in such a way that a woman with a clinical breast abnormality can have the clinical examination, the imaging (mammography and or ultra-sound scan) and the biopsy (core-cut and or cytology) carried out at the same visit. The diagnosis can be provided to the patient there and then and if cancer is confirmed, she can be put into the sympathetic hands of the clinical nurse specialist and her name placed on the list for the next MDT meeting. At that point a plan of action, that involves all the clinical disciplines, is agreed and the operation arranged at the patient's convenience; not as a surgical emergency. As well as humane, this approach together, with the introduction of adjuvant systemic therapy, has probably contributed to the encouraging fall in mortality since the mid 1980s.

Surgery for Breast Cancer: Less Is More

It has been a long and bitter struggle to complete the journey from the maximalist radical mastectomy plus radiotherapy (if you insisted on adding massive lymphoedema of the arm to the woman's burden), to the minimalist local excision, sentinel lymph node biopsy (SLNB) plus radiotherapy to the breast, as is our current default approach. Of course not all women are suitable for breast conserving surgery if the size of the cancer is large relative to the size of the breast or the cancer happens to be multifocal. In such cases developments in breast reconstruction or subcutaneous mastectomy with prosthetic implants, have displayed the ingenuity of my onco-plastic surgical colleagues who I have admired from afar, but that topic is a distraction from the main narrative.

I said that it was a "long and bitter struggle". The bigotry and hostility of the advocates of the radical approach had to be witnessed to be believed. Those of us in the front line were subjected to *ad hominum* attacks and publically accused of murdering women by neglect. Such dinosaurs were simply incapable of understanding the alternate model of the disease and we had to wait a long time for them to lose their influence and die off. As well as the bitterness, it was a long struggle because at each step of the way, clinical trials had to be carried out comparing more versus less surgery, to allow incremental progress. (Radical v. Modified Radical; Modified Radical v. Simple Mastectomy; Breast conserving surgery v. Mastectomy; Radical axillary dissection v. level I/II dissection; level I/II dissection versus SLNB). Each RCT required an infrastructure, thousands of selfless patient volunteers; and long enough follow up for sufficient "events" to accrue for the analysis of the primary outcomes measures: overall survival and disease free survival. For much of this we must acknowledge the innovative skills and clinical trials of Prof. Umberto Veronesi of the Institut Tumori, Milan [3] as well as Bernard Fisher and the NSABP. [4] At one point only Veronesi's group "overshot" in withholding radiotherapy altogether after tumourectomy, when the local recurrence rate was unacceptable. [5] This one step too far demonstrated the self-correcting nature of the scientific method. The other step too far, was a trial I was involved in comparing surgery plus tamoxifen with tamoxifen alone for the elderly. [6] From this we learnt the important lesson, that age alone is no reason for therapeutic compromise and that surgeons are better at achieving a "complete" local response than the medical oncologists!

References

[1] Fisher B, The surgical dilemma in the Primary Therapy of Invasive Breast Cancer: A critical appraisal. Chicago: Year Book Publishers (current Problems in Surgery), 1970.

[2] 'Sudden fall in breast cancer death rates in England & Wales', Beral V, Hermon C, Reeves G, Peto R,. *Lancet* 1995; 345:1642-3.

[3] Veronesi U, Saccozzi R, Del Vecchio M, et al Comparing radical mastectomy with quadrantectomy, axillary dissection, and radiotherapy in patients with small cancers of the breast. *New England Journal of Medicine* 1981; 305:6-11.

[4] Fisher B, Montague E, Redmond C et al, Comparison of radical mastectomy with alternative treatments for primary breast cancer. *Cancer* 1977; 39:2827-2839.

[5] Veronesi U, Luini A, Del Vecchio M, Greco M, Galimberti V, Merson M, et al. Radiotherapy after breast-preserving surgery in women with localized cancer of the breast. *N Engl J Med* 1993; 328(22): 1587-91.

[6] Fennessy M, Bates T, MacRae K, Riley D, Houghton J, Baum M. Late follow-up of a randomized trial of surgery plus tamoxifen versus tamoxifen alone in women aged over 70 years with operable breast cancer. Br J Surg. 2004 Jun;91(6):699-704.

Chapter 30

The Golden Ibex of Santorini: A Convergence of Cultures and Technologies

(The International Journal of Surgery
Volume 2, Issue 1, Pages 61 January–April, 2004)

3,600 years ago the Island of Santorini (Thera) blew its top. In the most cataclysmic volcanic eruption in the recorded history of our planet, 30 cubic kms of magma in the form of pumice and volcanic ash buried the Island and its civilisation. These dramatic events have given rise to a number of legends and myths. Firstly the destroyed civilisation of the Island of Strongili (as the Island was known before the eruption) gave rise to the legend of the lost City of Atlantis. The apparent sudden destruction of the Minoan civilisation on the Island of Crete used to be ascribed to this catastrophic event although modern day archaeologists no longer believe this to be true. Finally, the timing of the volcanic eruption was undoubtedly close to the timing of the exodus of the Jews from ancient Egypt and a rational explanation for the ten plagues described in the Old Testament follows some of the predicted events with a volcanic eruption of this magnitude. For example the column of ash above the volcano could produce a shadow long enough for the sun to be obliterated at noon over ancient Egypt. Furthermore the inflow of the Mediterranean Sea into the volcanic cavity followed by the tidal wave might have accounted for the dry crossing of the *Reed* Sea (? The Nile delta) by Moses and the children of Israel, followed by the destruction of Pharaoh and his legions shortly afterwards. Bible stories and legends of lost civilisations are beautiful but the reality might exceed the expectations of many sceptics.

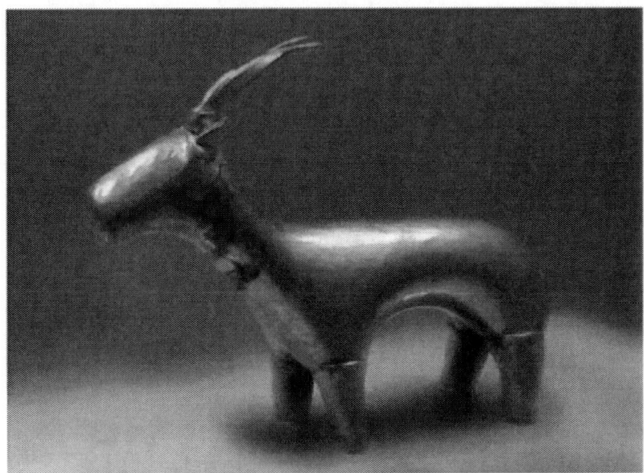

Golden Ibex of Santorini.

Approximately three years ago, a shaft was being dug to provide foundations for a permanent protective cover over the archaeological excavations at Akrotiri, a site at the southern tip of the crescent shaped island. Amongst the rubble, a workman discovered a perfectly preserved wooden box that was thought to serve some late Bronze Age domestic role. On opening the box, the archaeologists were both surprised and delighted to discover a most beautifully crafted and perfectly preserved Golden Ibex about the size of a newborn kitten. Closer inspection revealed that it was hollow with all four limbs welded at the junction with the trunk. The local experts assumed it was fabricated by using the lost wax technique, but the technique for welding the limbs onto the trunk was a mystery, as was its role within this lost Civilisation (See figure).

As an object this sublimely proportioned artefact can be looked upon in three ways. Firstly as an object venerated for its beauty and for all we know, venerated in its time as a household God, a pocket size adumbration of the Golden Calf worshipped by the children of Israel a few years after the exodus from Egypt. Secondly it could be looked upon as an archaeological curiosity capable of throwing light on the Bronze Age civilisations of the Cicladean Islands and their trading links with ancient Egypt to the South and the biblical Kingdoms to the East. Finally it was a technological challenge to assay the gold and interpret the technique for joining the limbs to the trunk that in its own way would shed light on its archaeological provenance.

In the last week of August 1997 a group of us assembled on the Island of Santorini as guests of Mr Peter Nomikos, the founder of Photoelectron Corporation for a scientific advisory Board meeting. I had been working with Photoelectron Corporation for about three years developing a technique for intra-operative radiotherapy in the treatment of early breast cancer using a miniature X-ray generating source developed by the Company. This device, about the size and the shape of a Gucci handbag, accelerates electrons down a metallic capillary tube that then hit a gold target generating soft X-rays from a point source at its tip. Introduced within the cavity following wide local excision of an early breast cancer it can deliver a full booster dose of radiation to the excision margins, (but that's another story). [1] The Nomikos Foundation also supports the archaeological explorations of Akrotiri and for that reason I was privileged to witness an historic first in the history of archaeology.

On Friday the 30th August a group consisting of archaeologists, technologists and oncologists gathered in the subterranean laboratories of the archaeological Museum in Thera. The Golden Ibex was placed upon a laboratory table and the miniature X-ray source was directed precisely at the weld at the junction between a hind limb and the trunk of this enigmatic beast. The device was switched on, electrons were accelerated down the capillary tube and X-rays from the gold target at the tip of the device excited the molecules within the Bronze Age weld of the ancient gold of the Ibex. The signal from the excitation of these molecules was then picked up by another extraordinary technological invention developed for the NASA Mars exploration project. This detection probe then provided us with a waveform printout describing the precise content of the solder. Thus with the benefits of modern technology the artisan of an ancient Cicladean culture was able to speak to us over the Centuries. It is difficult to describe the sense of awe we all experienced at this unique amalgam of art, archaeology, technology and the joker in the pack: clinical oncology! The results from this experiment were quite remarkable; the miniature electron generator has thrown new light on a lost civilisation and perhaps Atlantis is not a legend after-all.

The following day our celebrations were cut short when we learnt of the tragic death of Diana, Princess of Wales.

Reference

[1] Vaidya JS, Baum M, Tobias JS, A new technique for Intra-operative radiotherapy after breast conserving surgery. *Ann Oncol* 2001;12:1075-80.

Chapter 31

Intra-Operative Partial Breast Irradiation after Breast Conserving Surgery: The History and Outcomes of The TARGIT Trial May 2014

Dans les champs de l'observation le hasard ne favorise que les esprits préparés.
(In the fields of observation chance favours the prepared mind.
Louis Pasteur, Lecture, University of Lille, 7 December 1854)

I'm a great advocate of Pasteur's dictum shown above but I also believe that chance alone, as defined by synchronicity, also plays its part in the history of important scientific advances. Within a few days of returning from my visit to Santorini I greeted my new PhD student, Mr Jayant Vaidya (Jay). He had come to me with the highest recommendations from my old friend, Professor Indraneel Mittra (Neil), head of the breast cancer unit at the prestigious Tata Memorial hospital in Mumbai. The previous year, whilst working with Neil, Jay had published a very important paper in the British Journal of Surgery. [1] Many of the women attending the Tata Memorial hospital with early stages of breast cancer were subjected to a total mastectomy because they lived in rural areas and simply couldn't afford to hang around Mumbai for the six weeks necessary to complete radiotherapy to the residual breast tissue, had they have been offered the default treatment of breast conserving surgery as would have been the convention in the UK or USA.

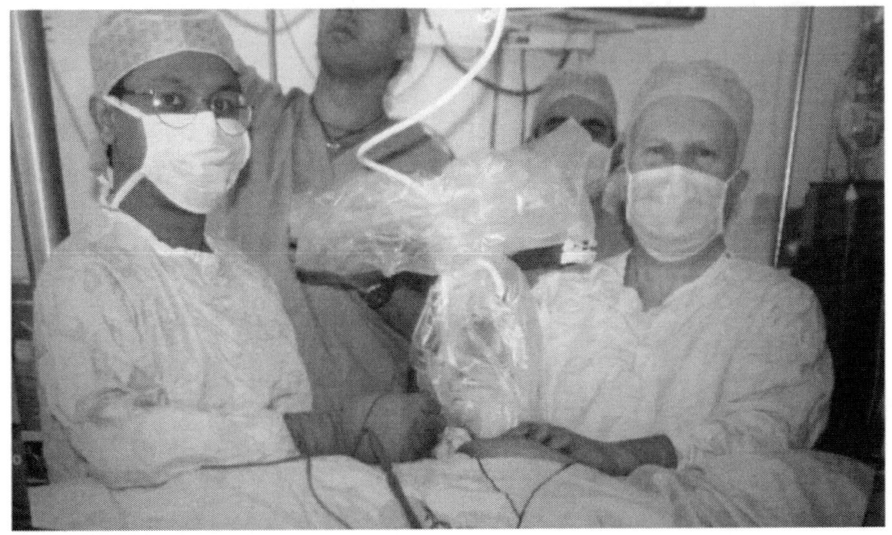

TARGIT first case 1998.

Jay went on to carry out whole organ analysis of the breast specimens, searching carefully for additional foci of breast cancer outside the confines of the obvious lump with which the primary cancer presented itself. He confirmed what others had described, that additional foci of disease were common, and this was the justification for whole breast radiotherapy after breast conservation. He even went further and used three-dimensional techniques for reconstructing the internal geometry of these additional occult foci of disease and reported that about 80% had more than one focus of disease and in about 60% of cases these additional occult lesions were distant to the "index quadrant" bearing the clinically obvious lump. These observations would convince most surgeons that whole breast radiotherapy was essential after "lumpectomy" and breast conserving techniques. However, as I was soon to learn, Jay was unlike *most* surgeons I had ever met; he was already exhibiting the early signs of progressive *scepticaemia.* Jay refused to accept the prevailing dogma that whole breast radiotherapy (WBRT) was mandated after lumpectomy by pointing out that in close to 100% of women who suffer a relapse in the breast; the local recurrence (LR) was in the index quadrant very close to the primary lesion. That simple observation provoked Jay, Neil and myself to publish a letter in the Lancet with the heretical suggestion that all these sub-clinical (occult) lesions found on whole organ analysis were not programmed to progress, or in other words might be considered "latent" rather than active pathology. [2] If such was the case then instead of 6 weeks of WBRT, we might be able to develop a new way of delivering radiotherapy at the time of surgery using the miniature electron/Xray generator invented by Alan Sliski and Ken Harte, working for Photo-Eletron Corp (PeC) and demonstrated to me on the Island of Santorini. We would call this partial breast intra-operative radiotherapy or IORT for short. A development like this might not only take the pressure off our radiotherapy centres but also more importantly, offer the prospect of breast conservation for women living more than 100 miles away from these centres; a particular boon for unfortunate women in the resource poor parts of the globe.

To begin with we had to recruit a radiotherapist who might share our vision. That proved easy as my close friend and colleague of over 20 years, professor Jeffrey Tobias (Jeff), shared my iconoclastic cast of mind. Next we needed a physicist and Jeff had no difficulty in finding a young Greek PhD student, Marinos Metaxas, who played the key role in monitoring doseimetry, quality control and safety.

The first tricky hurdle we had to overcome was the design of the applicator to fit over the Xray source. The electron generator accelerated the charged particles to hit a gold target that then emitted soft Xrays from a point source so as to produce a rapidly expanding spheroid of ionising radiation. This had to be contained so that the maximum dose would strike the cavity following the removal of the tumour together with a cuff of healthy tissue, whilst protecting normal tissue and the staff in the OR. As a start we made plaster casts of the tumour bed after lumpectomy in a number of cases and found that the shape of the cavity was impossible to mimic in the design of the applicator. We therefore decided on the elegant and simple solution of manufacturing as series of applicators with spheres of different diameters with the point source of the Xrays sitting at the epicentre of each of these spheres. We then prepared ourselves to fashion the cavity at the time of surgery so that it sat tightly opposed to the surface of the sphere, effectively conforming the geometry to the target to the beam, rather than the convention of conforming the shape of the beam to the target. Having got that far, the physics and engineering departments at the University, working closely with PeC, built a prototype gantry to hold the treatment unit steady in three-dimensional space for the 30-40 minutes estimated treatment time. I wont go into any of the details on all the technical work needed to calculate the dose and time of delivery but suffice it to say that our radiotherapy and radiobiology team concluded that using this 50 kV device we would need to deliver 20 Gy at the surface of the tumour bed that attenuated to 5-7Gy at 1.0 cm into the breast tissue. Having developed the technique, we had to seek ethical approval for a phase I/II trial in a small group of patient volunteers.

Our institutional ethical review body gave us approval for a trial of 20 patients providing they went on to have WBRT, they were enabled to give fully informed consent knowing that they were pioneers in an experimental treatment. We had no difficulty in recruiting our first few volunteers, as they and all subsequent patients seemed to grasp intuitively what we were trying to achieve (more than can be said about many clinical oncologists). Furthermore these patients had the added bonus of avoiding the last week of treatment after WBRT when conventionally the radiation oncologists delivers 5 days of boost therapy to the tumour bed. We were all ready to go when we hit the first set of buffers. The chief nurse of our operating theatres refused to allow us to use this new device in her OR suite as it might pose a threat to her staff. She remained adamant in spite of us trying to explain that the rapid attenuation of these soft X rays meant that virtually no X rays would escape the target area; further protection would be provided by tungsten impregnated drapes covering the body of the patient; and all the staff remaining in the OR during the time the X rays were being delivered would wear lead aprons and hide behind a lead screen. It was to no avail, so in the end the first three cases had to be done in the basement of the radiotherapy department under conditions somewhat reminiscent of a World War 1 front line dressing station.

The first case was scheduled for July 2nd 1998 and I couldn't sleep the night before, imagining all the things that could go wrong. We started on the dot of 08.30 am with Jay as my first assistant for the operation and Jeff and Marinos standing by monitoring the radiotherapy equipment. The removal of the tumour and surrounding tissues was easy but the dissection of the axillary lymph nodes was difficult because of the appalling lighting in the bunker. Once the surgery was complete we positioned a sterile 3.5 cm diameter applicator in the cavity and I prepared myself to tailor the healthy breast tissue to approximate to the surface of the plastic sphere. At that very moment ***the Hand of God*** intervened, or for the sake of my secular readers, "we got lucky", something no one could have predicted happened: the fatty breast tissue spontaneously adhered to the applicator surface by some kind of magical property of surface attraction. No tailoring was needed other than to reflect and retract the skin over the tumour bed well away from the neck of the applicator at the surface of the sphere. We then applied X ray sensors all around the field of surgery to judge the rate and distance of attenuation of the X ray dose, applied tungsten impregnated plastic sheets to the anterior surface of the patients body, positioned our anaesthetist and physicist behind a lead screen and then beat a retreat to the coffee room. There we met up with Peter Nomikos, CEO of Photoelectron Corp (PeC) who, unlike us had a major financial stake in the outcome of this case, and nervously drank our hospital ersatz coffee whilst making polite conversation. After about 45 minutes we were summoned back, rescrubbed and gowned, re-draped the patient and removed the applicator. The tumour bed was dry and healthy looking and that went for the anaesthetist and physicist. The wound was closed in the conventional way and stayed closed thereafter. The patient woke up with no problem and it was a close call as to who was most relieved as she was wheeled back to the ward. The X ray detectors remained un-fogged, confirming no escape of X rays from the treatment area.

We were quietly self-congratulatory, none of those American "high fives" in those days. In fact our behaviour was that of English gentlemen, although of those present one was Indian, two were Greek and Jeff and myself were only one generation English. I couldn't sleep again that night with the excitement of what we had achieved and the vistas of opportunity it opened.

The second case went equally well and in both cases the wounds looked perfectly healthy and remained closed after removing the sutures two weeks later. Paradoxically I was a little concerned that in both cases the wounds and the subcutaneous tissues felt so healthy that I began to doubt if we were actually delivering any radiotherapy at all. I learnt the truth the hard way with case number three. I must have got a little careless in closing the breast tissue around the neck of the applicator and accidentally caught the under surface of the skin in my purse string suture. This patient developed a small radiation burn the size of a dime (for my English readers that is a small coin worth 10 cents about the size of an old fashioned sixpenny piece.) Fortunately it healed spontaneously with no scarring.

Apart from this the first twenty cases went without mishap and the additional WBRT failed to add to any anticipated skin toxicity.

We continued to recruit into a pilot study and recorded details of toxicity and acceptability, but still added WBRT to the IORT in all cases. As we gained confidence with the technique we were delighted by the remarkably low toxicity of the treatment. At the same time we could describe a high level of acceptability by the patients. The full details of the methodology were published in 2001-2002 by which time we had coined the acronym TARGIT (targeted intra-operative radiotherapy) to describe the technique. [3, 4] In the fullness of time we recruited an unselected group of over three hundred cases that showed a remarkably low LR rate over a five year period, but that was of course outside a randomised controlled trial. Along the way our group, who now included a new member, professor Mohammed (Mo) Keshtgar (who took over from me as one of the surgeons in the team when I retired from the National Health Service), encountered cases who under normal circumstances would not have been suitable for WBRT for technical or medical reasons and would expect to be subjected to a mastectomy. We began to offer such women TARGIT "off protocol" most of whom leapt at the opportunity.

I'll never forget one such woman who had been blind since birth, who could not abide the thought of making the hazardous journey to a from the hospital five times a week for 6 weeks. Her first name was Rose and she was fiercely independent. She was also something of a clairvoyant. It was if with the loss of sight she had developed a 6th sense by way of compensation. She always knew it was me when I entered the room and she could also deduce my mood in an uncanny way. But there was one occasion when she tested my congenital scepticism to breaking point when she claimed that she had been communing with the spirit of my dead brother David. I'd never mentioned anything to her about my personal life let alone that my youngest brother who had died suddenly two years earlier. The message she carried beyond his grave made the bristles on the back of my neck stand on end as there was no one she might have encountered in her visits to the hospital who could have tipped her off that her visit coincided with David's birthday.

All such patients did well, at least in the short term, and this added to our confidence in launching the trial that we had been working towards after four years of preparation. For ethical reasons we decided to select a group of patients who were judged to have a low risk of LR and randomised them between IORT (TARGIT) and conventional WBRT. The exclusion factors included age below 45, large tumour size and other details of pathology that predicted a high risk of relapse within the breast. (I beg the indulgence of any specialists reading this essay as it is written for generalists and lay people. Full details are of course available in the references cited below) however I must emphasise from the start that there were two vital components in the design of the trial, (a third was to follow) that has led to much misunderstanding and frequent misrepresentation since the results were published. The first of these was that the design was "pragmatic" in other words reflecting the reality of clinical practice. This has always been our favoured approach because the results become generalizable in routine use. With the best will in the world and the best pathologists in the world, the initial biopsy of the tumour does not always accurately reflect the true pathological typing of the tumour. In about 15% of cases that look favourable when planning treatment after diagnosis, turn out to carry areas of pathological detail that changes their prognostic outlook. It was agreed therefore that these patients would go on to receive WBRT. In other words we were comparing two policies *not* two treatments; "one size fits all" WBRT with a risk adaptive policy of TARGIT + WBRT in about 15% of cases who we had misclassified after the initial biopsy. The patients were made aware of this possibility in the informed consent procedure.

The next important detail in the trial design was the issue of "non-inferiority".

Most clinical trials are designed to detect if the new treatment is better than the old treatment but the TARGIT trial was designed to show equivalence in outcome in terms of relapse in the conserved breast, on the reasonable assumption that our patients would prefer that their treatment was completed at the time of surgery without the need to return to the hospital five times a week for up to 6 weeks.

As you can never *prove* equivalence statistically, unless the total population is included in the trial, you have to determine the upper limit for the primary event analysis (LR in this case) beyond which non-inferiority can no longer be sustained. It sounds complex but in principle it quite an easy concept to grasp.

Various members of our group carried out patient preference studies (PPS) to determine at what level of risk of a local recurrence would the patient accept in order to enjoy the benefits of IORT and thus avoid the ordeal of up to six weeks of daily treatment, always assuming there was no additional risk of death from breast cancer. It turned out that the majority of women asked this question would settle at around the 2.5% level. After this the statistics get a bit difficult but in the end we felt confident that a trial with over 1,000 patients in each arm would be powerful enough to determine whether TARGIT was "non-inferior" or not. At the same time, we appointed an independent data monitoring committee with the authority to stop the trial if there was evidence that we had already crossed that threshold whilst recruiting or if there was a worrying trend for an excess death rate in one or other arm of the trial. I hope by now that my intelligent lay readers can at least understand the principles of a non-inferiority trial but sadly to this day many medically qualified critics cannot grasp this simple principle.

We launched the trial early in 2000 after registering the protocol with the Lancet and satisfied the institutional ethical review bodies. We started slowly and with some trepidation but to our delight most of the patients we approached to volunteer for the trial, were quick to understand and happy to take part. The main rate-limiting factor was the fact that we were a single centre trial dependent on one prototype machine. In due course the engineers at PeC came up with a more robust and sensible design for the assembly holding the electron generator. This gantry was mobile so that in theory the unit could be moved from one OR to another but apart from that we were in a "catch 22" situation. PeC couldn't sell their devices until we had the results of a trial demonstrating the safety and efficacy of TARGIT but it would take forever for us to recruit 2,000 patients to prove the point. For this reason the trial took off very slowly. Sadly PeC went into receivership in 2002 and we thought that our pioneering work was all for nothing. Just when we had abandoned hope a new player appeared on the scene. Karl Zeiss, the famous German lens and optical device company, decided to buy up the patents and assembly line for the manufacture of the TARGIT equipment, which they named as INTRABEAM, and the whole endeavour was charged with new energy and enthusiasm.

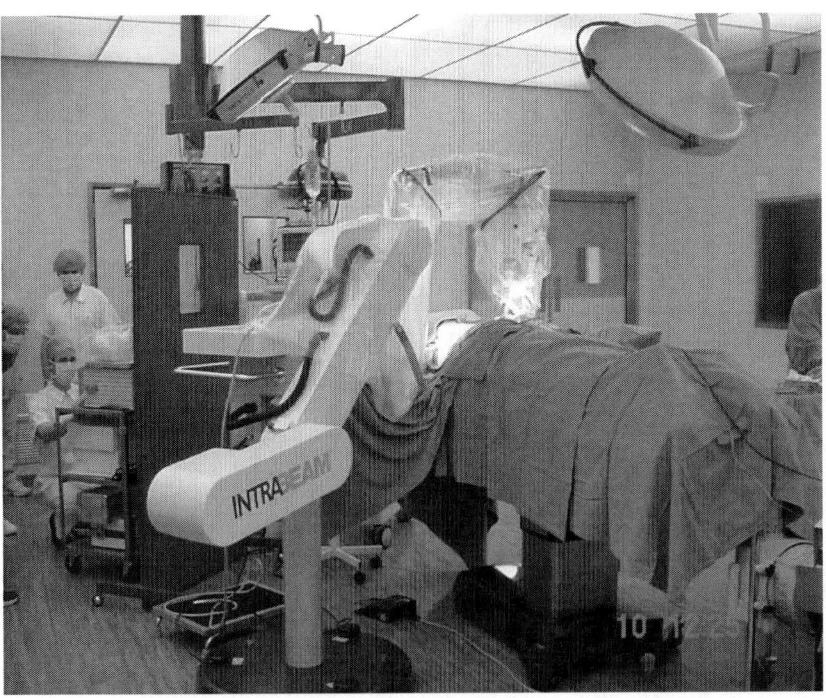

INTRABEAM in action 2012.

For a start they provided a system for the Department of Radiation Oncology in Mannheim linked to the University of Heidelberg, headed up by Professor Frederik Wenz. He became a major asset for the team, not just because we had another centre recruiting but also because Professor Wenz was a world authority on radiation biology. Very rapidly he recalculated the dose and duration of treatment based on the latest in vitro and in vivo methodology and discovered that we had again got lucky, in that our earliest calculations weren't far out from the optimum dose and duration of therapy according to the volume of breast tissue irradiated. He was vocal in his support for the methodology and published widely in the radiotherapy journals providing much needed expert endorsement for TARGIT. [5]

The next major centre to join us was in 2004, lead by Professor David Joseph in Perth Australia in collaboration with their new professor of surgery, Christobel Saunders, who just happened to be one of my protégés from UCL where she had completed her higher degree under my supervision. Along with a professor of radiotherapy and a newly minted professor of surgery we were also very lucky to recruit Max Bulsara, a world-class statistician. Because of the extreme difference in time zones Max was often called upon to work all round the clock whenever the pressure was on. Never once did he complain. This welcome addition to the family came at a cost that could only be judged in retrospect. Australia is a huge country and many of their population live in remote townships in the "outback" up to 1,000 miles away from a major medical centre. Women in these areas would have their breast lumps removed by general surgeons and once cancer was diagnosed, they were flown in to the nearest oncology centre. It made sense therefore for our collaborators to modify the protocol for practical reasons.

Patients were only accepted for the TARGIT trial if there was a rim of healthy tissue surrounding the margins of the excised tumours as well as fulfilling all the entry criteria for a low risk group. Only then would they receive the intra-operative radiotherapy as a second surgical procedure up to a month after the original surgery. These protocol revisions were so significant as to amount to a different trial for two reasons. Firstly they were a better-selected group of low risk cases and secondly the intra-operative treatment was delayed and we couldn't predict how this might play out in the long run. We therefore elected to describe the Perth cohort as the "post pathology" group with the original design of the trial now being described as the "pre-pathology" group. This new cohort were treated as a new stratum nested within the main trial with its own randomisation allocation allowing us to analyze the whole population and the two strata separately because of the *a priori* reasoning, that the outcomes might be different, although we couldn't guess which way the dice would fall. I will return to this matter later on in this story.

In 2005 the radiotherapy centre in Aviano serving the Veneto region of North East Italy joined in, headed up by professor Samuelle Massarut (another protégé of mine) As well as rapidly adding to the recruitment of patients, this group were ultimately to provide some original biological insights that accounted for the counter-intuitive results when the trial was finally published (*vide infra*). The next major milestone was the recruitment from two oncology centres in Copenhagen, during the year 2007. Their effort was lead by a very tall and handsome Danish gentleman, Henrik Flyger. Because the trial was recruiting from two competing oncology centres covering the whole of the city, and they had only one set of INTRABEAM equipment, they elected to join with Perth using the post pathology protocol. The Danish group recruited patients at such a speed they soon overtook all other centres, some of whom had been entering patients for more than 5 years. This was both a blessing and a curse because although it helped us to reach our final target accrual it also meant that the average follow up of cases was diluted; the faster we recruited the shorter the median follow up became. This matter came back to haunt us once we were ready to publish, another matter I shall return to shortly.

Finally it is worthy of note that during the years 2005-2007 we were able to recruit centres in California under the charismatic leadership of Professor Laura Esserman from the University of California San Francisco together with her second in command Michael Alvarado.

At long last, 10 years from the start, we finished recruitment to the trial with 2,232 patients from 28 centres in 9 countries in April 2010. This was just in time for us to present our preliminary results at the American Society of Clinical Oncology (ASCO) that was to be held in Chicago in May that year. Now ASCO is big, very big. It's considered the most important "cancer fest" in the calendar, attracting more than 40,000 delegates each year with huge competition to present new data from the world of cancer research. We assumed that the first results from the TARGIT trial would be of such great interest that our paper would be a sure-fire hit for a presentation at a plenary session before the whole assembly. In the end we had to satisfy ourselves with a poster presentation in a small back room. I confess to feeling humiliated by standing in front of the poster that summarized our results waiting for the odd passer by to stop and listen to my pitch.

The results were very clear even though we acknowledged that the median follow up was short for reasons explained above. Taking the whole cohort (pre and post pathology) the local recurrence rate (LR) was 1.2% in the TARGIT arm of the trial and 0.95% for those treated with conventional whole breast irradiation (WBRT). These were very low rates of LR by any comparisons with the past confirming our selection criteria of low risk were correct. Furthermore, these rates of LR were almost equivalent and well within the non-inferiority boundary.

The novel therapy was very well tolerated with 1.9% wound complications for TARGIT and 1.3% for WBRT. When it came to significant radiotherapy damage TARGIT actually performed better (0.54% v 2.1%)

There was some media interest in the UK following our press release but little in the USA so overall it seemed to float like a lead balloon.

In spite of that my spirits rose after I embarked on a nation wide lecture tour organised by Karl Zeiss that took me to centres in Florida, Texas, California, Virginia, New York and Washington. I delivered my lecture to 24 different audiences and was on the whole well received, but then most of my American colleagues are very polite. The warmest reception I received was in San Francisco where the breast cancer unit had already determined to make TARGIT available as standard of care in low risk patients. This enthusiasm reflected the concerns of their patients who lived on the wrong side of the Bay Bridge, who couldn't tolerate the conventional 22 daily visits to UCSF on the West side due to the perpetual traffic jams.

Without doubt the most interesting of my visits was the last one where I ended up at the HQ of Medicare just outside Washington. The word had got back to them from ASCO, that some "limey" had spoken about a new radiotherapy technique for breast cancer that was not only equivalent to conventional treatment and better tolerated by the patients, but was actually a damn sight cheaper, something never heard of in the annals of oncology of the USA! I was therefore summoned to appear before a high-ranking panel that determined what new technology might be allowed into the basket of treatments for patients unable to afford private care. The fact that this coincided with the launch of "Obamacare" might have had something to do with this last minute invitation. Again I was very well received and the panel was extremely polite in their expert cross-examination. For reasons beyond my ken some of the panel wore beautifully pressed army uniform almost as if I was up before a court marshal. At the end, the chairman summed up in my favour and announced that this was amongst the best data ever presented to his committee and the only problem remaining was how I might persuade American radiation oncologists, who were paid for each treatment, to accept that all the patient needed would be one shot instead of 22 fractions. I agreed that if adopted it would indeed lead to severe pain in their wallets but that wasn't my problem as we had a National Health Service free at the time of delivery. Those smug words would return to haunt me over the next four years.

Unlike British clinicians, those from the USA see no shame in being paid a fair rate for the job or looking upon their medical practices as business opportunities.

Within about 18 months of our presentation at ASCO followed almost synchronously by a publication in the Lancet, [6] my colleagues in America had figured out business plans with TARGIT as a "loss leader" and ultimately a reasonable reimbursement scheme based on outcome rather than number of interventions. INTRABEAM sales in America have taken off whilst here in the UK as I write in May 2014 we are still waiting for the National Institute for Clinical Excellence (NICE) to pronounce before TARGIT can be made available in the NHS. So far there are only 6 centres in the NHS offering this service and two in the private sector throughout the whole of the UK.

Returning to the summer of 2010, I now reconvened the TARGIT working party to plan the way forward. We agreed that the results so far confirmed the safety of the technique but were a little premature as a test for efficacy because of the limited follow up of the last 1,000 patients to be recruited. So it was decided to wait a couple more years for the study to mature. In addition we predicted that a second look at the data in 2012 would allow for enough local recurrences to have accumulated, sufficient to look at the pre and post pathology strata separately.

At this point I made another serious error in judgement. Many of our participants wanted to continue randomizing new patients as they remained in "equipoise"; others wanted to continue recruiting to complete "sub-protocols" relating to quality of life and cardio-toxicity, whilst others who had not yet joined the trial wanted to jump on the train before it left the platform. The net result of this was that we recruited another 1,200 patients in two years who added little by way of new "events" (i.e. local recurrence) yet diluted the median follow up further so that it remained more or less the same as at the initial publication!

Parking that aside for the moment, this new analysis produced remarkable results that stirred up a controversy that will run and run.

At this point I would like to summarize our results as they were presented by Jay Vaidya at the San Antonia Breast Cancer Symposium (SABCS) in December 2012 and later published on line in the Lancet in November 2013.

The SABCS is an unusual gathering that for historical reasons has become the biggest breast cancer specific meeting in the world in spite of the fact that it is based in a corner of Texas inaccessible by direct flights from the UK. It is always held in the week before Christmas promising mild and sunny weather whilst also promising severe snowstorms over Chicago that nearly always paralyzes the American domestic air services when you try to fly home. San Antonio is famous for the Alamo and Davey Crocket. The Alamo is quite under-whelming even at the first visit and Davey Crocket wore a hat made from a gutted beaver and invented the Bowie knife before crossing a red line in the sand or something like that. It is also famous for the Alamo, sorry I've already said that but best of all is Dirty Dick's a restaurant on the River Walk which is famous for it's beef ribs in BBQ sauce served by very rude waiters. The River Walk is also quite famous for being a walk along a river that has a number of Mexican restaurants as well as Dirty Dick's. As you may note after so many visits I'm suffering from San Antonio fatigue. Anyway during SABCS week I recognize more people on the street at any time than I do in my hometown London that is famous for err, lots of stuff.

Irony aside it is the best meeting if not the biggest meeting in the world for folk like me and was the best showcase for the updated results of TARGIT and on this occasion we did get a plenary slot for Jay to deliver a 10 minute talk that in no way could do justice the complexity of the results.

The TARGIT Results

I want to summarize the outcomes starting with the simple things first.

The total cohort by this time numbered 3451 patients equally divided between TARGIT and WBRT. This group had a median follow up of only 2 years and 4 months. Had we stopped recruiting in 2010, the original cohort of 2232 would have had a median follow up of 3 years 7 months. In retrospect we already had an answer with the first 1222 patients who by now had a median follow up of "the magic" 5 years. (I'll return to that point shortly)

Within the total cohort we had two strata for *a priori* analysis, 2298 in the original pre-pathology protocol and 1153 in the nested stratum using the post-pathology protocol (mostly Perth and Copenhagen). These numbers are substantial when compared to trials of radiotherapy in the past.

The first thing to say is that with increasing numbers and more than 1,000 cases with a median follow up of 5 years the safety and toxicity was excellent in both arms of the trial with the TARGIT group doing a little better than its comparator.

Next it is worth pointing out that deaths from breast cancer were exceptionally low in both arms, 2.6% for TARGIT and 1.9% for WBRT. This shouldn't be too surprising as about two thirds of patients in the trial were screen detected and based on current opinion; about half of these would have been over-diagnosed. [8]

So far so easy, but I now want to discuss the results for the primary end point in the trial, local recurrence in the breast (LR), and the secondary end point, overall survival (OS) i.e. deaths from all causes. For each of these end points I will structure the results for the three groups, first the combined cohort (A+B), second the pre-pathology stratum (A) and thirdly the post pathology stratum (B).

To make it understood at a glance, I include a table showing the results in a 3x2 matrix giving the point estimate and confidence intervals in brackets. (For the statistically minded of you these are Kaplan Meier 5 year estimates and for those suffering with OCD check out details in references 6 and 7)

	LR		OS	
	TARGIT	**WBRT**	**TARGIT**	**WBRT**
A+B	3.3% (2.1-5.1)	1.3% (0.7-2.5)	3.9% (2.7-5.8)	5.3% (3.9-7.3)
A	2.1% (1.1-4.2)	1.1% (0.5-2.5)	4.6% (1.8-6.0)	6.9% (4.3-9.6)
B	5.4% (3.0-9.7)	1.7% (0.6-4.9)	2.8% (1.3-5.9)	2.3% (1.0-5.2)

From this we can deduce that the combined analysis shows a small numerical excess of LR in the TARGIT arm that remains within the non-inferiority boundaries. For OS there is a small excess with WBRT that is not significantly different. However when considering non breast cancer deaths, there were only 17 in the TARGIT arm and 35 in the WBRT arm. This difference was marginally significant and resulted from an excess of cardiovascular deaths and other cancers. The net effect in absolute terms ended up as 12 more LR and 14 fewer deaths comparing the novel therapy with the conventional approach. I concede that this is difficult to accept and might yet turn out to be the play of chance linked to a small number of events; yet at the very least we can safely claim that we had demonstrated *non-inferiority* for the secondary outcome measures.

In the pre-pathology stratum LR is comfortably within the non-inferiority boundary with an absolute difference of 1.0% against the upper limit preset at 2.5%. The net effect in this stratum was 4 more LR against 13 fewer deaths.

In the post-pathology arm there is an excess of LR in the TARGIT group, in absolute terms 3.7%, that therefore fails the non-inferiority test. OS in this stratum was very close with only 0.5% difference. Again expressed in absolute numbers there were 8 more LR against one less death.

(For those who wish to check out the workings of these analyses that justify my conclusions, please read the Lancet paper published in print in February 2014) [7]

The reaction to these results by our critics has been one of fury and at times coming close to accusations of scientific misconduct. Our response to these expressions of disbelief have by now been recorded in the correspondence columns of the Lancet and our explanation for the excess occurrence of non breast cancer deaths following whole breast radiotherapy can be read in the Lancet paper of March 2014 [7] and other supportive studies concerning the toxic effects of whole breast radiotherapy. [9,10,11,12,13,14]

Putting all that aside, and before I return to my summing up, I wish to identify a signal that's been lost in the background noise. Whether you love or hate our trial, hidden within the results of this huge clinical experiment is the proof of principle. The trial was predicated on the hypothesis that only a small fraction of those microscopic foci of malign looking pathology outside the narrow confines of the clinically apparent disease have the potential to progress into an invasive and life threatening disease if left untreated. I now wish to share with you some as yet unpublished data that strongly endorses this belief.

Using the mature cohort of 2232 patients I identified 737 cases in the pre-pathology stratum who received IORT alone without additional WBRT according to the TARGIT protocol. Based on the early work by Vaidya using whole organ analysis, 464 of these cases would have additional foci of disease with 370 of these foci being outside the index quadrant and outside the field of treatment offered by INTRABEAM. [1] Many of these patients would have been treated up to 10 years earlier yet at the time of analysis there have been 7 local recurrences in the index quadrant of the primary tumour together with 6 new primary tumours in the opposite breast. In the meantime, only two local recurrences (new primary tumours) have appeared outside the index quadrant in the breast with the presenting disease. This is not only proof of principle but probably the best evidence yet concerning the natural history of sub-clinical disease detected by mammography.

In other words this is the first prospective study supporting the concept of "over-diagnosis": the central concern in the screening controversy that will be addressed in the next section of this book.

Conclusion

For the remainder of this essay I want to express my personal take away message from these complex results and how they may be applied to current practice. But first a declaration of potential conflict of interest is in order. I have a huge intellectual investment in the outcome of the TARGIT trial, not to mention the countless hours of hard graft and diplomacy to see it through to the end. It would therefore be inevitable for me to put a spin on the results to show them in a favourable light. When I started out working with PeC on the prototype and early stages of the trial I was awarded share options but sadly, when the company collapsed, I lost that financial incentive, nor do I have any patent rights. However, along the way Karl Zeiss has been generous in funding my travels and offering me consultancy fees and honoraria for speaking at meetings that promote INTRABEAM, but even that source of income has now dried up. So judge me as you choose, but this is where I stand.

Firstly I believe the data ***are*** mature because however you calculate the median follow up you cannot ignore the fact that the peak incidence for local recurrence is at two to three years after surgery ***not*** five years which is a "magic number" derived from counting the fingers on one hand. [15]

Secondly I believe the results are better than expected and that the timing of the intra-operative radiotherapy is critical, not simply because the novel therapy is better at killing neighbouring cancer cells in the tumour bed, but because of recent observations that TARGIT perturbs the contents of the "cytokine soup" in the tissue fluid in the tumour cavity in such a way as to abrogate the local environment, that in normal circumstances acts as a favourable culture medium for residual or circulating cancer cells. [16] In other words, TARGIT doesn't just kill cells by radiation but changes the microenvironment that normally provides a comfortable nest for cancer cells to grow.

Given that, I have little difficulty in making a recommendation. If the patient fits the entry criteria of the trial and if the risk adaptive approach is implemented, then I can see no reason to deny that woman the TARGIT approach so that she can avoid up to 6 weeks traipsing back and forward to the radiotherapy centre. At the same time in many geographical areas of the resource poor and even resource rich part of the world, patients can even avoid the mutilation of a total mastectomy. Even if you can't accept the favourable difference in all cause mortality you can at least accept that non-inferiority has been established in the pre-pathology stratum at no cost in additional toxicity and even, as it transpired, an improved cosmetic outcome. [17]

References

[1] Vaidya JS, Vyas JJ, Chinoy RF, et al. Multicentricity of breast cancer: whole-organ analysis and clinical implications. *Br J Cancer* 1996;74(5):820-4.

[2] Baum M, Vaidya JS, Mittra I. Multicentricity and recurrence of breast cancer. *Lancet* 1997;349(9046):208.

[3] Vaidya JS, Baum M, Tobias JS, D'Souza DP, Naidu SV, Morgan S, Metaxas M, Harte KJ, Sliski AP, Thomson E. Targeted intra-operative radiotherapy (Targit): an innovative method of treatment for early breast cancer. Ann Oncol. 2001 Aug;12(8):1075-80. PubMed PMID: 11583188.

[4] Vaidya JS, Baum M, Tobias JS, et al. The novel technique of delivering targeted intraoperative radiotherapy (Targit) for early breast cancer. *Eur J Surg Oncol* 2002;28(4):447-54.

[5] Herskind C, Griebel J, Kraus-Tiefenbacher U, Wenz F. Sphere of equivalence--a novel target volume concept for intraoperative radiotherapy using low-energy X rays. Int J Radiat Oncol Biol Phys. 2008 Dec 1;72(5):1575-81. doi: 10.1016/j.ijrobp.2008.08.009. PubMed PMID: 19028280

[6] Vaidya JS, Joseph DJ, Tobias JS, Bulsara M, Wenz F, Saunders C, Alvarado M, Flyger HL, Massarut S, Eiermann W, Keshtgar M, Dewar J, Kraus-Tiefenbacher U, Sütterlin M, Esserman L, Holtveg HM, Roncadin M, Pigorsch S, Metaxas M, Falzon M, Matthews A, Corica T, Williams NR, Baum M. Targeted intraoperative radiotherapy versus whole breast radiotherapy for breast cancer (TARGIT-A trial): an international, prospective, randomised, non-inferiority phase 3 trial. *Lancet.* 2010 Jul 10;376(9735):91-102

[7] Vaidya JS, Wenz F, Bulsara M, Tobias JS, Joseph DJ, Keshtgar M, Flyger HL, Massarut S, Alvarado M, Saunders C, Eiermann W, Metaxas M, Sperk E, Sütterlin M, Brown D, Esserman L, Roncadin M, Thompson A, Dewar JA, Holtveg HM, Pigorsch S, Falzon M, Harris E, Matthews A, Brew-Graves C, Potyka I, Corica T, Williams NR, Baum M; TARGIT trialists' group. Risk-adapted targeted intraoperative

radiotherapy versus whole-breast radiotherapy for breast cancer: 5-year results for local control and overall survival from the TARGIT-A randomised trial. *Lancet.* 2014 Feb 15;383(9917):603-13. doi: 10.1016/S0140-6736(13)61950-9. Epub 2013 Nov 11. PubMed PMID: 24224997.

[8] Jørgensen KJ, Gøtzsche PC. Overdiagnosis in publicly organised mammography screening programmes: systematic review of incidence trends. *BMJ* 2009;338-341.

[9] Clarke M, Collins R, Darby S, Davies C, Elphinstone P, Evans E, et al. Effects of radiotherapy and of differences in the extent of surgery for early breast cancer on local recurrence and 15-year survival: an overview of the randomised trials. *Lancet* 2005; 366:2087-106.

[10] Darby SC, Ewertz M, McGale P, Bennet AM, Blom-Goldman U, BrØnnum D, et al, Risk of Ischemic Heart disease in Women after Radiotherapy for Breast Cancer. *N Engl J Med* 2013; 368: 987-998.

[11] Nilsson G, Holmberg L, Garmo H, Terent A and Blomquist C. Increased incidence of stroke in women with breast cancer. *European journal of Cancer* 2005; 41: 423-429.

[12] Nilsson G, Holmberg L, Garmo H, Terent A and Blomquist C. Radiation to supraclavicular and internal mammary nodes in breast cancer increases the risk of stroke. *British Journal of Cancer* 2009; 100: 811-816.

[13] Voskoboynik M, Urban P, Mileshkin L. Early cardiovascular deaths in patients with cancer. *N.Engl J Med* 2012; 367:1572-3.

[14] 15. Baum M, Chaplain M, Anderson A, Douek M, Vaidya JS. Does breast cancer exist in a state of chaos? *Eur J Cancer* 1999; **35**: 886–91.

[15] 16. Belletti B, Vaidya JS, D'Andrea S, et al. Targeted intraoperative radiotherapy impairs the stimulation of breast cancer cell proliferation and invasion caused by surgical wounding. *Clin Cancer Res* 2008;14(5):1325-32.

[16] 17. Keshtgar MR, Williams NR, Bulsara M, Saunders C, Flyger H, Cardoso JS, Corica T, Bentzon N, Michalopoulos NV, Joseph DJ. Objective assessment of cosmetic outcome after targeted intraoperative radiotherapy in breast cancer: results from a randomised controlled trial. *Breast Cancer Res Treat.* 2013 Aug;140(3):519-25. doi: 10.1007/s10549-013-2641-8. Epub 2013 Jul 23. PubMed PMID: 23877341

Chapter 32

The Historical and Cultural Determinants in the Evolution of Adjuvant Endocrine Therapy: Two Hemispheres Separated by A Common Language

(Commentary for Oncology 26:6; Jun pg 559, 2012)

There are historical and cultural differences between Europe and the USA that determined the direction of research into the adjuvant systemic therapy for breast cancer. As is often the case, the truth eventually came to rest somewhere in the mid- Atlantic; not sunk like the Titanic 100 years ago, but cruising in ever decreasing circles, not quite sure in which direction it should sail next.

George Beatson, a Scottish surgeon working in Glasgow, in 1896, described the first systemic therapy for breast cancer. [1] That of course was surgical castration at a time when hormones had yet to be discovered. He got lucky and was right for the wrong reasons. The first trials of adjuvant ovarian ablation were carried out in Manchester and Norway about 60 years later. [2,3]

Prior to the discovery of tamoxifen by Walpole in the late 1960s [4] the only endocrine therapies were surgical (or radiation) ablation of the ovaries, the adrenal glands and the pituitary gland. As these modalities were controlled by surgeons (initially including radiotherapy), the tradition has been for surgeons in the United Kingdom, to take the lead in this subject. In addition, the most important endocrine therapies that replaced the removal of the ovaries, and the barbarity of adrenalectomy and hypophysectomy i.e. tamoxifen, anastrozole and the LHRH agonist goserilin, were British inventions of the scientists working or ICI (later Astra Zeneca). [4,5,6] It is not surprising therefore, that at least in one area, Europe lead America. (I can't help myself in remarking that parts of this history have been rewritten and the first ever RCT showing the advantage of adjuvant tamoxifen [7] almost never appears in American literature).

On the other hand, the whole conceptual revolution and the gestation of a research programme that continues to flourish after nearly 50 years of endeavour, is thanks to one American visionary, Bernie Fisher from Pittsburgh PA. [8] Furthermore whilst medical oncology as a speciality languished like a Cinderella in the UK, the subject took off like a rocket in the USA as the Nixon cancer plan of 1971 tried to outdo the Kennedy NASA programme that lead to the first lunar landing three years earlier. It is no surprise therefore that the Americans with a little help from our friends in Milan [9] lead the way in pioneering adjuvant chemotherapy.

Although ultimately this twin track approach was a great success, in the early days it actually acted as a barrier to progress.

If you'll forgive the cultural stereotyping for a moment, the American frontier spirit (no gain without pain; the bigger the better) resulted in dismissing soft option remedies like hormone therapy advocated by the decadent Europeans, in favour of big complex stuff that at one time lead to the abomination of high dose chemotherapy and bone marrow grafting (the less said about that the better). However, just focussing on adjuvant endocrine therapy for a moment, there was also a subtler fall out that has yet to be adequately resolved.

In this very comprehensive review, the authors start the section on the management of pre-menopausal women as follows:

> "The ASCO guidelines published in 2010 recommend tamoxifen for premenopausal women….. They state that, currently, the benefit of ovarian suppression is not known….".

What? Still not known after more than 40 years of effort; how can that be?

I believe there are two reasons to explain this paradox. Firstly the early trials in Manchester, Oslo and Edinburgh, were hopelessly underpowered.

[2,3,10] Furthermore they were hampered by the failure to stratify cases by ER status in the era prior to the description of the hormone receptor mechanisms. By the time we woke up to the importance of power and the beta error, and before patients in trials of endocrine modalities were selected by ER status, the chemotherapy battalions were off and conquering the world. Without question, adjuvant chemotherapy offers the best chance yet for many younger women with early breast cancer, but it also has the unfortunate (or maybe fortunate) side effect of rendering these women amenorrhoeaic. [11] There can be little doubt that part of the benefit of adjuvant chemotherapy for the younger women is mediated by a chemical ovarian suppression. From the first EBCTCG overview in 1985 [12] until this day we are trying to untangle this knotty issue. At times the debate was acrimonious and almost lead to a new Anglo-American war of independence (this time the Anglos wanted independence from the Yankies), but now is all sweetness and light as many multinational groups are finally working together to resolve the problem once and for all.

The situation with tamoxifen however is clear. Assuming the patient's tumour is HR+, then both pre and post menopausal women benefit and within reason the longer their exposure, the better although 5 years is a reasonable compromise. [13] I also think that the absolute risk of endometrial cancer has been exaggerated because of ascertainment bias. Most women on tamoxifen develop sub-endometrial oedema that on ultrasound scanning can't be easily distinguished from endometrial thickening. [14] This then leads to endometrial biopsy and the occasional random detection of early endometrial cancer (EC). Remembering that most symptomatic cases of EC are cured by hysterectomy, my advice would be not to monitor the poor woman's womb even if there is reimbursement for this futile activity! Many women complain of hot flushes on tamoxifen, but close examination suggests that in many cases the problem is the withdrawal of the concomitant prescription of HRT or the onset of the menopause provoked by the diagnosis and treatment of the breast cancer.

Coming now to the aromatase inhibitors (AIs) I share the view that they demonstrate a class effect although there is a tantalizing suggestion that the steroidal AI, exemestane has a slightly different spectrum of activity to the two non-steroidal drugs, anastrozole and letrozole. [15]

The AIs are only active in postmenopausal women (and even judging that status can be tricky in the peri-menopausal period) so it was reasonable to conduct trials on pre-menopausal women combining ovarian suppression with an LHRH agonist and an AI, but the results so far are a little disappointing.

In contrast, the trials comparing monotherapy with tamoxifen or an AI have produced an unequivocal answer with a small (approx 3%) absolute improvement in disease free survival. [16] As the original PI of the ATAC trial I can speak with some authority on the subject. Because of the favourable side effect profile of anastrozole, the ATAC study was powered up for "non-inferiority" so we considered the improved outcome in DFS an added bonus. I remain disappointed that the improvement in DFS has yet to be translated into a gain in overall survival. Having lived with the data since 2001, I have a hunch why this might be.

There are many elderly women in the ATAC trial, some even recruited in their 80s and recent papers have shown that the older patients are at diagnosis, the more likely they are to die of co-morbidities. [17] I believe this might dilute out a real survival advantage for, say, the under 65s, and I hope that the guardians of the data set might get round to looking at that possibility. The side effects of polyarthralgia can be severe in a small percent of cases but the problem of loss of bone mineral density is relatively easy to manage. After all we don't avoid the use of cytotoxic drugs for fear of bone marrow suppression we merely monitor the patient's WBCC. The same approach should apply to women taking an AI, who need regular bone mineral density scans.

In many ways the advent of adjuvant systemic therapy can be considered one of the greatest advances in the history of cancer therapy.

Mortality from breast cancer has been falling rapidly since the publication of the first EBCTG overview in 1988 [12] and it is estimated that close on two thirds of this decline relates to the rapid adoption of adjuvant endocrine therapy.

Envoi

It is said that 50% of the global expenditure on cancer treatment occurs in the USA a country that carries only 5% of the global tumour burden. Anti-American rhetoric would have it that US hegemony and solipsist attitudes have lead to more and more expensive therapies that are unaffordable in resource poor countries. I would argue that the USA is the global engine and powerhouse that has kept the pharmaceutical industry in business and indirectly paid for the salaries of most of the best basic scientists in drug discovery programmes throughout the world.

Patents aren't forever. Tamoxifen is now widely available as cheap and effective generics and anastrozole, I believe, will also be out of patent soon.

With that, effective endocrine therapy should become affordable in the developing world that carries the greatest tumour burden and the two hemispheres of the resource rich countries can take pride in that.

So in which direction should this good ship sail in the future? Mechanisms of endocrine resistance amongst HR+ tumours are under intense scrutiny but it shouldn't beyond the wit of man to engineer the conversion of HR- tumours into HR+ phenotypes. It's quite simple really. Just get the pluri-potential stem cells in the cancer to repopulate the tumour with ER +ve cells. [18]

References

[1] Beatson GT, On the treatment of inoperable cases of carcinoma of the mamma: Suggcstions for a ncw mcthod of trcatmcnt, with illustrativc cases, *Lancet* 1896; ii:104–107.

[2] Patterson R, Russell MH. Clinical trials in malignant disease. Part II. Breast cancer: value of irradiation of the ovaries. *Journal of the Faculty of Radiologists* 1959; 10:130–145.

[3] Suppression of ovarian function in primary breast cancer. Nissen-Meyer R *Acta Radiologica* 1965; 259(Suppl):

[4] Harper MJK, Walpole AL. Nature 1967; 212:000–000. Walpole AL. *Journal of Reproduction and Fertility* 1968; 3(Suppl 4): 000–000.

[5] Yates RA, Dowsett M, Fisher GV *et al.* Arimidex (ZD1033): a selective, potent inhibitor of aromatase in post-menopausal female volunteers. *Br J Cancer* 1996;73:543–548.

[6] Nicholson RJ, Finney EJ, Maynard PV. Activity of a new analogue of luteinising releasing hormone analogue, ICI 118,630, on the growth of rat mammary tumours. *Journal of Endocrinology* 1976; 79:51–52.

[7] Baum M, Brinkley DM, Dossett JA, et al. Controlled trial of tamoxifen as adjuvant agent in management of early breast cancer: Interim analysis at four years by the Nolvadex Adjuvant Trial Organization *Lancet* 1983; 5th Feb:257–261.

[8] Fisher B. The surgical dilemma in the primary therapy of invasive breast cancer: A critical appraisal. Chicago: Year book publishers (current problems in surgery) 1970.

[9] Bonadonna G. Brusamolino E, Valagussa P, et al. Combination chemotherapy as an adjuvant treatment in operable breast cancer. *New England Journal of Medicine* 1976; 294: 405-410.

[10] Adjuvant ovarian ablation versus CMF chemotherapy in premenopausal women with pathological stage II breast cancer: The Scottish trial Scottish Cancer Trials Breast Group and ICRF Breast Unit, Guy's Hospital London, *Lancet* 1993; 341:1293–1298.

[11] Rose DP, Davis TE. Ovarian function in women receiving chemotherapy for breast cancer. *Lancet* 1977; ii:1174–1176.

[12] Effects of adjuvant tamoxifen and of cytotoxic therapy on mortality in early breast cancer. An overview of 61 randomized trials among 28 896 women. Early Breast Cancer Trialists' Collaborative Group (EBCTG) *New England Journal of Medicine* 1988; 319:1681–1692.

[13] Fisher B, Dignam J, Bryant J, et al. Five versus more than five years of tamoxifen therapy for breast cancer patients with negative lymph nodes and estrogen receptor-positive tumors. *J Natl Cancer Inst* 1996;88:1529–42.

[14] The ATAC ('Arimidex', Tamoxifen, Alone or in Combination) Trial: Transvaginal ultrasound scan findings overestimate observed pathological findings in postmenopausal gynaecologically asymptomatic women before treatment. Jackson TL, Duffy SRG. *Breast Cancer Res Treat* 64 (Suppl 1), 64, Abs. 2000.

[15] Smith, I. E. and M. Dowsett (2003). "Aromatase inhibitors in breast cancer" N Engl J Med 348: 2413-244 [19] Anastrozole alone or in combination with tamoxifen versus tamoxifen alone for adjuvant treatment of postmenopausal women with early breast cancer: first results of the ATAC randomised trial The ATAC Trialist's Group *Lancet* 2002; 359:2131–39.

[16] Thurlimann B, Keshaviah A, Coates AS, et al. for the Breast International Group (BIG) 1-98 Collaborative Group. A comparison of letrozole and tamoxifen in postmenopausal women with early breast cancer. *N Engl J Med* 2005;353:2747–57.

[17] Schairer, C., P.J. Mink, L. Carroll, et al., *Probabilities of death from breast cancer and other causes among female breast cancer patients. J Natl Cancer* Inst, 2004. 96(17): p. 1311-21.

[18] BRCA1 - Conductor of the Breast Stem Cell Orchestra: The Role of BRCA1 in Mammary Gland Development and Identification of Cell of Origin of BRCA1 Mutant Breast Cancer. Buckley NE, Mullan PB. Stem Cell Rev. 2012 Mar 17. [Epub ahead of print]

Chapter 33

A Tyranny of Cheerfulness: Pink Ribbons at the Human Rights Watch Film Festival 29th March 2012

(Film review for Spiked On-line)

What about my human rights, eh!? I was the one forced to watch a feature length documentary consisting mostly of wobbly women dressed in pink Lycra cat suits jumping up and down and joyfully screaming yee haw: If they weren't just jumping up and down, they were marching, jogging, skydiving or marketing cute teddy bears, balloons and that protean manifestation of breast cancer awareness-the twist of pink ribbon. Yes folks, this is how they mark breast cancer awareness month in North America and it's not a pretty sight.

In the UK it tends to be a little more restrained, genteel and dignified, but to me, breast cancer awareness month has always been "Black October". That's the month when our breast clinics become overloaded with anxious young women who have been coerced into breast self examination (BSE) and, as might be expected in women below the age of the menopause, have noticed some lumpiness in the top left hand corner of their left breast. BSE is a thoroughly bad idea and has long been condemned by the cognoscenti as causing more harm than good.

So who on earth is responsible for this annual breast fest? Well it just happens to be the cosmetic industry, Avon and Estée Lauder, aided and abetted by the Komen Foundation, or maybe the other way round. One would be unkind to suggest that for the most part the organizers weren't acting in good faith and the participants weren't well meaning if naïve, but golly gosh it's an awfully good show for product placement. At the merchandise booths around the start and finishing lines of the mini marathons or the "I'm walking backwards for breast cancer challenge", you'll find all your groceries, toys, fashion items, bling and even automobiles in shocking pink. The price might be a little inflated but the extra goes to breast cancer research, so everyone is a winner. If you eat 12 cartons of some expensive branded yoghurt and send the lids to somewhere, someone will donate a dime to the pink charity.

If you shop using AMEX that month, then any item you buy will end up with a cent donated to the cause. And what is that cause? Why, it's the war against breast cancer.

Cut to the "Stage 4 Breast Cancer Support Group"

Leaving irony aside for a moment these scenes contained genuine pathos. Groups of women getting together in the privacy of someone's parlor, had one thing in common, they had been diagnosed with stage 4 disease and as one bitterly commented, "there ain't no stage 5". All of them complained that they'd done everything right, had no family history, checked and screened themselves with evangelical enthusiasm, ate 5 portions a day, run mini marathons, fought the good fight and yet here they were knocking at death's door. Their anger and frustration was palpable and justified. They will not be one of the "survivors", so somehow they will end up being judged and found wanting. So where, they ask, do all these millions of pink dollars go to and why are we still dying of breast cancer?

Cut to Talking Head

As a welcome break to this tyranny of pink joyfulness and optimism, the film was punctuated by interviews with grayish, serious "experts", who included the odd apologist PR person from the cosmetic industry. All these grave faces, apart from the smooth Avon man, poured scorn on the failure of the pink ribbon campaign and questioned how these millions of dollars were spent. Me too. I can recall most of the important advances in the diagnosis and management of breast cancer in the last 40 years and they were mostly funded by the NCI and more recently the Department of Defense in the USA, the MRC and CRUK (CRC+ICRF) in the UK, and the pharmaceutical industry worldwide. I cannot recall any examples of game changing work funded by the pink dollars. I could be wrong and would be happy to stand corrected.

The film should have stopped at that point but no, at last we were getting to the whole point of the story: it's another conspiracy theory, another Michael Moore moment.

There has been a 30% increase in the incidence of breast cancer in the last 30 years and yet only 5% of NCI money goes on prevention research. The subject is certainly worthy of a greater investment but not for the reasons suggested in "Pink Ribbons".

Apparently many cosmetic products contain carcinogens so it's all about a cynical conspiracy of the hypocritical cosmetic industry to distract the gullible public from the real cause of this increase in incidence. I have little time for some of the claims made by the cosmetic industry, particularly for products that have "clinically proven" that creams in pink jars are capable of increasing the collagen content of the skin so that you stay looking younger for longer or even worse those that claim to get rid of "cellulite". But to claim that cosmetics also cause breast cancer whilst tightening your booty, is a bit too far fetched. Cosmetics have always been with us even from the time of Ancient Rome, so can hardly account for the recent sudden surge in the incidence of breast cancer. Yet we don't have to look far for the real culprits, they are staring at us in the face. Now here we come to the delicious irony that from time to time makes life worth living: it's breast cancer awareness campaigns themselves that are guilty of producing this pseudo-epidemic. Think Pink means more screening mammograms at younger ages. More screening means more over-diagnosis and that means more mastectomies. Further data confirming this phenomenon emerging from Harvard University, was published this week in the Annals of Internal Medicine and featured on the BBC website http://www.bbc.co.uk/news/health-17585735 and the Daily Telegraph's as well.

http://www.telegraph.co.uk/health/healthnews/9181445/Breast-cancer-screening-resulting-in-unnecessary-treatment.html

If we stopped screening today the incidence of breast cancer would fall at a stroke by about 25%. That's the conspiracy. I suspect that the Pink Ribbon brigade is in league with the screening industry and that much of their research money funds the development of imaging technology of ever increasing sensitivity and the lobbying government agencies. In support of these unkind thoughts I came across this report from the Wall Street Journal published in January 2010.

> "One of the largest breast-cancer-awareness groups, Susan G. Komen for the Cure.... turned to GE in October (breast cancer awareness month) when it lit the Great Pyramids pink to mark a major screening initiative in Egypt. Neither GE nor the Komen group would say how much the event cost. In 2007, GE sold limited edition pink cameras to Home Shopping Network, which donated a portion of the sales to Komen. Imaging and film companies whose products go into mammography equipment have made pink DVD players, pink computer flash drives and pink cell phones, a portion of whose sales raise money for Komen and other breast-cancer groups. In events at the Capitol, Komen for the Cure founder Nancy Brinker has praised GE's digital mammography technology, and she received a public-service award from the company."
>
> http://online.wsj.com/article/SB126325763413725559.html
> www.djreprints.com

There is often a synchronicity of unrelated events in my life that add to my self-delusion that I am someone's pawn in some grand eternal plan. At lunchtime on the same day of the premier of "Pink Ribbons", I attended the first meeting of the panel given the task of rewriting the leaflet that will accompany future invitations for breast cancer screening in the NHS. Professor Amanda Ramirez, Professor of Liaison Psychiatry at Kings College London, chairs this committee. The committee is independent of the one chaired by Professor Sir Michael Marmot, that is currently reviewing the future of breast cancer screening in the UK and both will report to the department of health later this year. If nothing else our new information leaflet will describe the harms as well as benefits of screening in absolute rather than relative numbers. Faced with the knowledge that screening is associated with the over-diagnosis of cancer, many women will make the legitimate decision not to accept the invitation. I therefore prophesy that the incidence of breast cancer in this country will fall whilst that in the USA will continue to rise.

To paraphrase the immortal words of Eartha Kitt:

> A beauty spot may cost a lot,
> But pink I think is more expensive.

Screening for Breast Cancer

Preface

This section requires a preface of its own for reasons that will soon become clear.

I've learnt to my cost over the last decade or so, that whenever I write or speak about population based screening for breast cancer by mammography I have to start with this disclaimer:

I have devoted my life to improving women's health and I have been driven in part by the bad family history of breast cancer.

I am one of the architects of the British National Health Service Breast Screening Program (NHSBSP) and understand the theory and process of screening.

I have already justified the first clause in my disclaimer in the previous sections of this collection of essays but I now need to explain the paradox how in good faith I set up the service for the NHSBSP in the South East of England in 1998 and since then become one of the most vociferous proponents for closing it down.

In 1987 the Forrest report was published just two weeks before a general election called by Margaret Thatcher, it having sat on her desk for six months. (1) This report was based on the review of all the available evidence that included two randomized trials plus three case control studies that predicted a 25% relative risk reduction in breast cancer (cause specific) mortality favoring those who were invited to screening. It is noteworthy that little space was allocated to the potential harms of population based screening by mammography.

Not surprisingly, the Thatcher lead government of the day, two weeks before a general election, endorsed the recommendations and promised that if re-elected a comprehensive screening program involving women 50-65 who would be invited every three years for mammography, would be established. The NHSBSP was to be rolled out across the UK between 1988 and 1990. The service would be based on fixed screening units close to population of high density and mobile units for remote areas. All of these district units would feed into a select group of regional specialist centers in major hospitals who would be provided with additional facilities and manpower to handle the predicted surge in activity following the first round of screening. At that time I was professor of surgery at Kings College Hospital, a major teaching hospital in South East London caring for a socially deprived population.

I was given the task, in partnership with Dr. Heather Nunnerly head of the imaging department, of setting up the first district unit in the South East of England. This unit was created in a small shopping mall called Butterfly Walk in Camberwell close to Kings College Hospital. Butterfly Walk takes its name from the "Camberwell Beauty" a species of butterfly that is now extinct, killed off by the urbanization and lead pollution from the exhaust pipes of the constant traffic jam that circles the erstwhile Camberwell "Green". All the mammogram reporting and subsequent clinical management would feed into the specialist breast cancer centre funded to support the NHSBSP. Kings College Hospital was one of the first of its kind in the UK. We were also given the task of setting up the training centre for all the clinicians, radiologists and radiographers who would staff the other units serving the South East of England as the program was rolled out. We were given 12 months to finish the job that was completed on time and on budget in spite of continuing with our full time day jobs. In the summer of 1988, the attractive and flamboyant Edwina Currie, minister of health in the new conservative government, formally opened the unit on Butterfly Walk. In a blaze of media attention the lovely Edwina, accompanied by the Mayor and other local dignitaries, cut the pink ribbon and wandered round the unit whilst Heather and I stood in the background completely ignored. In her words addressed to the BBC reporter and cameraman, Ms Currie explained how this new initiative would prevent breast cancer by catching it early so women would stop dying of the disease and that was proof enough that the National Health Service was safe in the hands of the Conservative party (or words to that effect).

Forgetting the snub, I was proud of what we had achieved and in good faith, accepting the evidence available at that juncture. I threw myself into my leadership role in the NHSBSP and was rewarded by being offered a seat on the National committee running the show.

My love affair with the NHSBSP was short lived. Unlike most of the other members of the National Committee, I was directly involved in the day to day care of those women referred on to me as a consequence of the activities on the front line of the screening program. I found it very distressing to have to cope with otherwise well women who had popped into the screening unit for a mammogram at the invitation of the Department of Health (DoH) whilst doing their grocery shopping in Butterfly Walk and then found themselves labeled as a cancer victim. Worst of all were the unexpected high numbers diagnosed with duct carcinoma in situ (DCIS), a condition we rarely saw before screening began. Many of these cases were multifocal and ended up with a mastectomy. How do you explain to a woman that she is "lucky" that we caught it early yet ends up having a mastectomy? None of the DoH staffers or public health specialists on the National committee had to face the reality of these heart-breaking interviews. We were soon to learn that 20% of the cancers diagnosed in Butterfly Walk were DCIS, yet before we opened our doors they amounted to less than 1.0% of our practice. I drew short term comfort from this observation assuming that in the fullness of time this initial peak in the incidence of DCIS would be followed by a fall in the incidence of invasive breast cancer. I couldn't have been more wrong as you will learn in the essays to follow.

In the early years of the service as we were building up our expertise and confidence we had to deal with the poor women who suffered false alarms. These were the ones with suspicious findings on the mammograms that lead to a biopsy that proved in the end to be benign. The waiting time for admission and biopsy and then the result of the pathology must have been agonizing for these women who were of the generation lead to believe that breast cancer was a fatal disease.

Within a few more years others noted that the "interval cancer" rates were far too high to achieve the predicted 25% reduction in cause specific mortality. "Interval cancers" are those that appear as clinically detected lumps in the intervals between two invitations for screening examination. These tend to be the fast growing tumors that slip through the net. It rapidly became clear to me that we would never meet our targets and also there was no evidence for the predicted fall of invasive cancers following the mopping up of all these cases of DCIS. Furthermore, updated analyses of the evidence in the Forrest report together with the publication of new trial reports, persuaded independent authorities to lower the estimate for the reduction in breast cancer mortality in a population based screening program from 25% to 15%. [2] After six or seven years into the program, by which time it had been rolled out to the four corners of the UK, including the Islands and Highlands of Scotland, it became obvious to me that the benefits of screening had been grossly overestimated whilst the downside had been virtually ignored. Yet the letter inviting women into the NHSBSP remained unchanged, optimistic, pretty pink and frankly coercive.

Things came to a head for me in December 1994. The deputy chief medical officer called an emergency meeting of the NHSBSP national steering committee in the week between Christmas and the New Year. The meeting was set up in order to come up with a strategy to protect the program in the face of the accumulation of adverse publications in the medical media (none of this had so far spilled over into the popular press). I argued passionately for a revision of the false promises in the leaflet that went out with the invitations so that the lay public would at least be able to make an informed choice, as in my mind it was a pretty close call to judge whether the benefits outweighed the harm. I was a lone voice at the table and the chairman summed up the opinion of the gathering as follows; "Professor Baum, if we include all this new information in the leaflets then the women are unlikely to attend and we will fail to reach our target of 70% uptake." To which I replied; "If that is indeed the view of this committee then I can no longer serve as I believe that women have the right to self determination, I hereby resign and intend to make my feelings felt but going public on the topic". True to my word I published a long letter in the Lancet entitled "Screening for breast cancer; time to think and stop", a few months later. [3]

The agents of the state responded with fury, and making use of their unlimited resources, sent glossy brochures to every doctor in the land that amongst other things ridiculed my stand. The leaflet went a little too far when they showed a graph describing a fall in mortality rates for breast cancer that they claimed was the result of screening. This was frankly fraudulent as they had frame shifted the curve to the right when in fact mortality rates had been falling since 1985, 3 years *before* Butterfly Walk was opened-thanks to the impact of the world overview of adjuvant systemic therapy. [4] I pointed this out but there never was a retraction or an apology.

25 years after the NHSBP was launched, the DoH was at last forced to set up an independent review that considered the adverse effects of screening; and to accept that women should no longer be denied the facts in helping them to

decide whether or not to accept the call that was to be rewritten as an invitation and not like a ***summons.*** [5]

References

[1] Forrest P, Breast Cancer Screening Report to the Health Ministers of England, Wales, Scotland and Northern Ireland, 1986.

[2] U.S. Preventive Services Task Force. Screening for Breast Cancer: Recommendations and Rationale. *Ann Intern Med* 2002;137: 344-6.

[3] Baum M. Screening for breast cancer, time to think-and stop? *Lancet* 1995; 346: 436-437.

[4] Burton RC, Bell RJ, Thiagarajah G, Stevenson C. Adjuvant therapy, not mammographic screening, accounts for most of the observed breast cancer specific mortality reductions in Australian women since the national screening program began in 1991. *Breast Cancer Res Treat.* 2012; 131(3): 949-55.

[5] Independent UK Panel on Breast Cancer Screening. The benefits and harms of breast cancer screening: an independent review. *Lancet* 2012; 380:1778-86.

Chapter 34

Breast Cancer Awareness Month: "Black October"

(Spiked on-line Jan. 2004)

Public Perception of Risk

Each year we enjoy breast cancer awareness month or what I choose to call "Black October". Each October women are advised to practice breast self-examination (BSE), a thoroughly discredited practice, and reminded that their risk of developing the disease is 1 in 11.

This number is true only if a woman outlives all competing risks to reach the age of 85, with 25 out of 26 women dying of other causes. It is essential therefore that both doctors and the lay public understand the risk of developing breast cancer in the age groups invited for screening and understand the expectation of life after the diagnosis of breast cancer in the absence of screening in order to appreciate the absolute value of submitting themselves to screening.

However before we get into that I wish to describe some of the biases inherent in mammographic screening which support my somewhat counter-intuitive view that screening ain't all that it's cracked up to be.

Biases in Screening

- **Lead Time Bias:** Say you get on a train to Edinburgh that crashes at Newcastle then the duration of your fatal journey depends on your departure point. If you leave from Milton Keynes your expectation of survival is two and a half hours whereas if you leave from Kings Cross it is three hours but you still die at the same time. In other words merely shifting the period of observation of breast cancer to the left might extend survival from the point of diagnosis without necessarily extending the duration of your life.
- **Length bias:** Say you trawl the sea for fish with a slow boat you'll catch the slow fish but miss those who can out swim your trawler. In other words, if you trawl the female population for breast cancer at intervals you will catch the slow growing cancers that might be cured if allowed to grow to a clinically detectable stage whilst missing the rapidly growing cancers that appear in the intervals between screening and are probably the ones that will kill you in any case.
- **Class bias:** Not all women invited for screening are "compliant" and graciously accept your invitation. The well-mannered upper classes who are health conscious tend to accept, whilst the ill mannered lower classes may ignore your invitation or never get it in the first place because they maybe of no fixed abode. Furthermore we know that the outcome of treatment stage for stage is better amongst the better off, so the apparent benefit of screening might just be a surrogate for class.

To get round these biases in order to truly assess the value of screening it is necessary to carry out randomized trial in whole populations with the outcome measure being breast cancer mortality.

The Trials of Screening and Relative Risk Reductions

There have been eight randomized or quasi- randomized trials of population mammographic screening for breast cancer. In addition, there have been a number of attempts to conduct a meta-analysis of all these studies to improve the precision of the estimate. [1,2] Finally there was the Cochrane review, which attempted to weight the studies for quality before providing a summary statistic. Let us first dispose of the latter, published by Olsen and Gotzche in the Lancet in 2001. [3] This provoked the editor of the Lancet,

Richard Horton to state, "At present there is no reliable evidence from large randomized trials to support mammography programs". [4]

Whatever the merits or flaws in the Cochrane review there are a number of unassailable facts that emerge. The Canadian study, that produced a negative result, was the only one with individual randomization with informed consent. The HIP study New York, which produced the most favorable result, excluded 336 subjects in the control arm because of a past history of breast cancer compared with 853 in the screened population. The Edinburgh trial, which randomized according to postal district, ended up with huge imbalances in socio-economic factors favoring those invited for screening. Finally the largest effects were seen in the trials with the worst equipment and the longest screening intervals.

We therefore start off with the concern that screening has no proven effect.

Let's leave that for a moment and consider the more optimistic estimates produced by two other overview analyses, the Swedish study [1] and the US Preventive Services Task Force 2002 [2]. Neither could show a significant advantage for women under the age of 50 (in fact the latest result from the Canadian trial for the <50 group actually showed a detriment for the first 10 years [5]) whereas their estimates for the >50 age group varied between a hazard ratio of about 0.75 (i.e. a relative risk reduction of 25%) and a hazard ratio of 0.84 (i.e. relative risk reduction of 16%) for breast cancer specific mortality. Let us now compute what that means in absolute terms so that an individual woman can work out her chances of benefit following a decade of mammographic screening.

The risk of a woman aged 50-60 for developing breast cancer is 2/1,000 a year or 2% over a decade (20 out of 1,000). The anticipated 10-year survival for clinically detected breast cancer in the absence of screening today is about 75%. Therefore we can expect 5 deaths per thousand women from breast cancer over this period (75% of 20).

The relative risk reduction for screening applies to these 5 women. From the above, a realistic estimate would be the saving of 1 life (a relative risk reduction of between 16 and 25%) after a decade of screening 1,000 women over the age of 50, whilst 999 have to share the cost and by this I don't mean financial cost but the price in terms of "side effects". [6]

The Down Side of Screening

Like any other imperfect screening tool there has to be a balance between sensitivity and specificity. Sensitivity is a measure of the ability to detect those cancers present in the population whereas specificity is a measure of the accuracy of the screening tool. These two measures tend to pull in opposite directions. For 100% sensitivity i.e. not missing a single cancer, specificity will fall and many women with benign changes on mammography will be recalled for biopsy. There always has to be a delicate balance between these opposing needs, to catch all the cancers whilst protecting women without cancer from false alarms and unnecessary invasive procedures. Even at it's best, for every cancer detected another woman will have a false alarm. Whereas at its worst, fuelled by a fear of litigation, the cumulative risk of a false alarm over a decade of screening is around 40%. [7]

All this unnecessary surgery not only has its morbidity but also tends to throw up pathology of borderline significance. The lay public can be forgiven in thinking that a pathologist can make a clear distinction between cancer and non -cancer, but sadly that is not the case. There is a whole spectrum of ranging from epithelial hyperplasia with or without atypia, lobular carcinoma in situ, low grade duct carcinoma in situ (DCIS), high grade DCIS, micro invasive DCIS and tubular carcinoma of uncertain significance and unknown natural history. A conservative estimate would suggest that less than half of these would threaten a woman's life if left undetected and yet they account for 20% of "cancers" detected at screening. [7] Furthermore many of these cases have field changes that effect the whole breast leading to a mastectomy for what might be a non- progressive condition. As a result the screening program ***cannot*** claim that there is a net reduction of the mastectomy rate in the population, the opposite might be the truth.

Next there is the issue of "lead time". If the woman with the screen detected cancer is either doomed to die or at the other extreme diagnosed with a cancer that would have cured if left to develop to the point of clinical diagnosis, she will live as a "breast cancer patient" for one or two years longer than needs be. Finally women invited for screening should be aware that the detection of DCIS with all the uncertainties described above might have an effect on the premiums for their health or life insurance.

Where Do We Go from Here?

I believe that to carry on complacently now that we know the full costs and benefits of screening is NOT an option. So what should be done? In an ideal world I would recommend that we shut down the service and divert the resources (opportunity costs) to other issues to preserve the health of women. This might include improving the clinical care of women with symptomatic breast cancer as, for example, getting rid of the 12- week waiting list in some parts of our country for postoperative radiotherapy. We could also fund first class breast cancer research with the £100,000,000 a year so released[1]. Prevention of heart disease and osteoporosis would save more lives than the prevention of breast cancer, [8] yet the strategies could well be the same with the use of selective oestrogen response modifiers (SERMS). However I see this as politically inexpedient so the best I could hope for here might be a shift in the screening window, to the 55-69 age group where sensitivity and specificity might be improved.

Finally, if nothing else, I believe there is an ethical imperative to offer women full informed consent with the harms and benefits spelled out in terms that don't patronize or deceive them. If, after that, the women vote with their feet-so be it. [9]

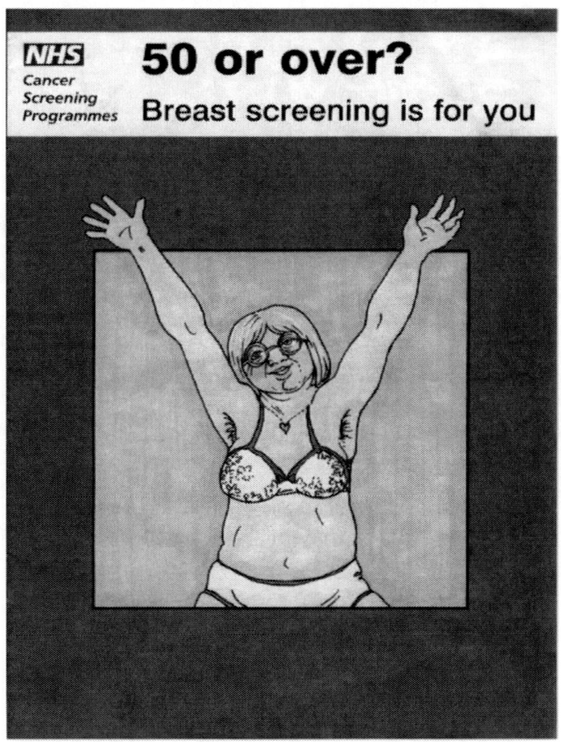

NHSBSP Leaflet inviting women with learning difficulties for screening.

References

[1] Humphrey LL, Helfand M, Benjamin KS, Chan MS, Woolf SH. Breast Cancer Screening: A Summary of the Evidence for the US Preventive Services Task Force. *Ann Intern Med.* 2002;137:347-360.

[2] Nystrom L, Andersson I, Bjurstam N et al. Long-term effects of mammography screening: updated overview of the Swedish randomised trials. *Lancet.* 2002;359:909-19.

[3] Ole Olsen, Peter C. Gotzche. Cochrane review on screening for breast cancer with mammography. *Lancet* 2001; 358: 1340-42.

[4] Horton, Richard. Screening mammography – an overview revisited. *Lancet* 2001; 358: 1284-85.

[5] 5.Miller AB, To T, Baines CJ, Wall C. The Canadian National Breast Screening Study-1: Breast Cancer Mortality after 11 to 16 Years of Follow-up. *Ann Intern Med.* 2002;137:305-312.

[6] Rembold CM, Number needed to screen: development of a statistic for disease screening. *BMJ* 1998;317: 307-12.

[7] Skrabanek P. Mass mammography. The time for reappraisal. *Int J Technol. Assess Health Care* 1989; 5: 423-430.

[8] Bunker JP, Houghton J and Baum M; "Putting the risk of breast cancer in perspective". BMJ, 1998; 317:1307–1309.

[9] Dixon-Woods M. Writing wrongs? An analysis of published discourses about the use of patient information leaflets. *Soc Sci Med* 2001; 52: 1417-1432.

Chapter 35

The Illusions and Delusions of Screening for Cancer

(Spiked April 2009)

"The largest threat posed by American medicine is that more and more of us are being drawn into the system not because of an epidemic of disease, but because of an epidemic of diagnoses. The real problem with the epidemic of diagnoses is that it leads to an epidemic of treatments. Not all treatments have important benefits, but almost all can have harms" [1]

Introduction

A couple of weeks ago I was showing off my newly acquired i-phone to my very bright 12-year-old granddaughter when she elected to "Google" my name. To my amazement the top hit appeared to link my name with that of Jade Goody. As far as I could recall I had never met with her, I have never knowingly watched Big Brother and I don't even research or treat cervical cancer. It appears that I was being stigmatized as the leading anti-screening dinosaur. Everything became clear when on Monday the 23rd March 2009, the Times published a full- page obituary on the short and tragic life of the reality TV celebrity, Jade Goody, whose dying wish was that women under the age of 25 should have access to screening for cervical cancer. The "Goody effect" has already provoked a campaign and a response from the Department of Health. I have nothing against the late Jade, in fact she reminded me of the type of patient that used to make my NHS clinics in central London such fun.

Nevertheless I feel the urge to defend myself and to explain why being a screening sceptic might after all place me on the side of the angels rather than to the darker side of Darth Vader. For a start I must hasten to mention that some of my best friends are women. My beloved mother died of breast cancer and my equally beloved sister is a long- term survivor of the disease. Galvanized by this experience I've devoted my whole professional life to fighting breast cancer, visualizing it as a slavering beast and in moments of self-delusion seeing myself as St. Michael. My wife's reminder, that this brand name is sewn in the back of my underpants, tends to bring me down to earth.

In addition I actually know a thing or two about screening. In 1987 when I was employed as Professor of Surgery at Kings College Hospital, I was commissioned by the DoH to establish the first breast-screening unit following the publication of the Forrest report. This unit was built near Camberwell Green in South East London and served as the training centre for the South-East of England.

Furthermore, for the last 8 years I've acted as the chairman of the National trial to evaluate PSA screening for the early detection of prostate cancer.

Suddenly, a confluence of events has thrown the subject of screening for cancer into the public eye again. To start with there was the publication of the Nordic Cochrane centre paper on mammographic screening in the BMJ in February 2009 [2], along with an open letter to the Times signed by me amongst 27 other experts, both of which provoked a debate on the wisdom of screening for breast cancer. Then there were two papers published in the New England Journal of Medicine in March, reporting on the early results of screening for prostate cancer by using the PSA blood test. [3,4] This was accompanied by banner headlines in the Daily Telegraph demanding PSA screening on the NHS that could save 2,000 lives a year. Later on I will explain just how wrong this statement was, but before then it behoves me to explain some of the delusions and illusions of screening in general.

> "For very complex problem there is a simple solution-and it's wrong" (H.L. Menken)

The majority of lay people could be forgiven for believing that one of the mainstays in the fight against cancer is "early detection". This belief has generated a European wide consensus that screening for cancer before it becomes symptomatic will save lives. It has also become the main plank in the government's campaign to improve cancer survival in the UK to match the highest levels achieved in the EU. In the vanguard of this campaign, the NHS screening programme for breast cancer (NHSBSP) by mammography has been lauded as a triumph and has laid claim to the responsibility for the dramatic decline in breast cancer mortality since its initiation more than 20 years ago. Those of us who have remained sceptical from the start have been branded as either misogynists or fools. Furthermore if its good enough for women, what about men's health as well? How can early detection of cancer be a bad thing? Although counterintuitive, a growing body of informed opinion is moving in that direction.

Biases of Screening That Can Disguise the Truth and the Diagnosis of "Pseudo-Cancers"

Let us start by considering two separate but related issues: firstly, biases of screening that give a false impression of benefit; and secondly, the over-detection of cancer "look-alikes" that if left undetected might never threaten a patient's life. The latter might even be described as catching the disease ***too*** early!

The *survival* from cancer is measured from the time of detection until recurrence and death. If a frame shift in the chronology of the disease due to screening occurs, then survival is automatically extended even if the ultimate outcome is the same; this is called lead-time bias. Of course if the "cancer" detected would never have threatened a woman's life in the first instance then that lead time might be as long as 30 years. Next, bearing in mind that the interval between screens is anything from one to three years, it is inevitable that the fast growing tumours with a bad prognosis will appear during the intervals, whilst the slow growing tumours with a good prognosis will sit around until found by mammography; this is called length bias. There is also another subtle bias that can be described as the "self selection" bias, in that women who accept invitations for screening might be demographically different to those who ignore the invitation. For a variety of reasons such women have better outcomes in the treatment of cancer, forgetting whether they were screen detected or not. The only way to account for these biases is to consider all the clinical trials of screening versus no screening and look for the pooled results described in terms of *mortality* i.e. the number of women dying in the screened group compared with those dying in the control group, rather than case survival. There is in fact a modest advantage to screening looked upon in those terms, as described in the recent publication in the BMJ: "Breast screening: the facts—or maybe not" by Peter C Gøtzsche and his colleagues from the influential and independent, Nordic Cochrane Centre. [2]

In this milestone paper they describe a synthesis of all the papers that describe both the benefits and harms of screening using absolute rather than relative numbers that make it easy for women to comprehend and conclude as follows. If 2000 women are screened regularly for 10 years, one will benefit from the screening, as she will avoid dying from breast cancer.

How does this equate with the promise of saving 1,400 lives a year described in the invitation to screening in the NHS leaflet "Breast Cancer The Facts"?

Well, in an attempt to figure this out I was lead on a paper trail from "Breast Cancer the Facts" to the NHS "Breast screening a pocket guide" to the report of the report of the Association of Breast Surgery at BASO June 2006 - at which point the trail went dead. However it is fairly simple mathematics to back calculate this number. At present there are about 12,000 deaths a year from breast cancer of which half would be in the age group screened. That would be in the region of 60,000 in a decade. 1,400 X 10 lives saved in a decade corresponds to roughly a 25% relative risk reduction; that is twice the rate that appears in the Cochrane report or for that matter in the US Preventive Services Task Force evaluation of the screening trials. [5] Looking at it another way, according to the 2008-year book of the Association of Breast Surgery at BASO, 16,000,000 have been screened over the last 10 years for the saving of 14,000 lives, giving a figure closer to 1 per 1,000 per decade who benefit from screening rather than 1 per 2,000 per decade as described in the Cochrane report. So it looks as if the NHS booklets exaggerate the benefits by a factor of two. I can't believe this is intentional; it's probably because those writing the leaflets haven't kept up to date. However even the 1:2,000 might be an over-estimate. Remember these data were derived from the trials that were mostly started in the 1970s and reported in the late 1980s. Since then, improvements in treatment, such as the adoption of tamoxifen and adjuvant chemotherapy, have narrowed the window of opportunity and we have witnessed a drop in mortality of 30%- 40% both in the age group that are invited for screening (>50) as well as for the younger woman. So perhaps the correct number might be 1:2,000 X 0.6, i.e.1:3,000

Forgetting the precise number, that one woman who benefits from a decade of screening has a life of infinite worth, and if screening were as non-toxic as wearing a seat belt, there would be no case to answer. However, there is a downside and that is the problem of the over-diagnosis of "pseudo-cancers". It is deduced by the Cochrane report that for every life saved,10 healthy women will, as a consequence, become cancer patients and will be treated unnecessarily. These women will have either a part of their breast or the whole breast removed, and they will often receive radiotherapy and sometimes chemotherapy. This is the tricky part of the story that is more or less denied by the screening fraternity and therefore deserves some close attention.

An Explanation for, and the Nature of, the over-Diagnosed Cancers

Screening for breast cancer is now adopted as an unequivocal good by most of the members of the EU. Invitations for screening promote this activity by being economical with the truth. [6] One of the uncomfortable truths concerns the over-diagnosis of both in-situ and invasive breast cancers in screening populations. [7] Over-diagnosis of breast cancer doesn't mean false positive rates; it means the detection and treatment of cancers that if left undetected would never threaten a woman's life and with which she would live, in blissful unawareness, until she died naturally of old age. We had always assumed that there was an over-diagnosis of duct carcinoma in-situ (DCIS), some of which had the potential of progressing to an invasive and life-threatening phenotype. However, there is now clear evidence that anything between 10% and 50% of invasive cancers detected and treated radically as a result of screening, would never threaten life. [8] As a result the overall mastectomy rate rises after any country implements screening, contrary to the implicit message in the NHSBSP leaflet, "Breast cancer the facts". [9]

How can this possibly be? Don't we know that if cancer is neglected it will progress to a life threatening condition?

By way of illumination let me propose that the pathological diagnosis of cancer at screening is based on a *syllogism;* (a *syllogism* is a logical argument in three propositions, two premises and a conclusion, the conclusion being specious). An easy to understand example of a syllogism runs like this. Vincent Van Gough was an artist. Van Gough is now judged as an artistic genius. Van Gough never sold a painting in his lifetime. Michael Baum is an artist, he has never sold a painting *ergo* he is a genius.

Cancer was defined by its microscopic appearance about two hundred years ago. The 19th century saw the birth of scientific oncology with the discovery and use of the modern microscope. Rudolf Virchow, often called the founder of cellular pathology, provided the scientific basis for the modern pathologic study of cancer. As earlier generations had correlated the autopsy findings observed with the unaided eye with the clinical course of cancer one hundred years earlier, so Virchow correlated the microscopic pathology of the disease.

However, the material they were studying came from the autopsy of patients *dying* from cancer. In the mid 19thC pathological correlations were performed on living subjects presenting with locally advanced or metastatic disease that almost always were pre-determined to die in the absence of effective therapy. Since then, without pause for thought, the microscopic identification of cancer according to these classic criteria has been associated with the assumed prognosis of a fatal disease if left untreated. The syllogism at the heart of the diagnosis of cancer therefore runs like this: people frequently die from malignant disease, under the microscope this malignant disease has many histological features we will call "cancer", *ergo* anything that looks like "cancer" under the microscope, will kill you. I would therefore like to argue that some of these earliest stages of "cancer" if left unperturbed, would not progress to a disease with lethal potential. These "pseudo-cancers" might have microscopic similarity to true cancers but these appearances are only a necessary rather than sufficient condition for a fatal disease. I would also like to suggest that many of the "risk factors" for the development of cancer are in fact the promotional agents of a latent condition that Welch has described as pseudo-cancers. If we stand back and take a broader look at nature this shouldn't be surprising. Conventional mathematical models of cancer growth are linear or logarithmic-more appropriate for the internal combustion engine than the exquisite organization of cell proliferation.

Most natural biological mechanisms are non-linear or better described according to chaos theory. The beauty of the tree in full leaf is because of its fractal geometry that looks remarkably similar to the microscopic appearance of the mammary ducts and lobules under the microscope. The rate of growth and the development of the lung or the fingers and toes in the foetus cannot be described in linear terms. Wound healing starts with the knife and ends when it needs to, although rarely wound healing carries on too long to leave an ugly keloid scar. Prolonged latency followed by catastrophe should not be all that surprising. We accept the case for prostate cancer, as we know that most elderly men will die with prostate cancer in situ and not of prostate cancer that has invaded. In fact, the UK national PSA screening trial is predicated on that fact with two a priori outcome measures defined: deaths from prostate cancer versus the number of cancers treated unnecessarily. Why oh why does the breast cancer lobby remain in denial? Of course now that the cat is out the bag they will have no choice but to include this fact in their invitations in order to avoid litigation from an irate woman in the future. Furthermore "the sins of the mother are visited on the daughter". We now have cases of women with screen detected DCIS whose daughters have had problems raising mortgages when the insurers have discovered this family history of breast cancer! [10, 11] However even their concession on this fact, as reported in the Times, only acknowledges one cancer over-diagnosed for every life saved. How on earth do they derive that number? The Cochrane report is transparent on this matter and the numbers are there for all to see. They simply record the numbers of breast cancers that have appeared in the screened group (observed) and subtract the numbers expected as seen in the unscreened control populations in the trials that have now been followed up for the majority of these women's lifetimes. (Observed-expected = over-diagnosis) How the DoH arrived at the figure of one to one is therefore inexplicable. The charitable conclusion is that they were caught off guard and trotted out the figures that are 10 years out of date rather than being guilty of a "dodgy dossier".

Prostate Cancer

By way of a minor diversion I want briefly to mention prostate cancer screening. In my preamble I mentioned the banner headlines in one of our respected broadsheets following the publications in the New England Journal of Medicine in March 2009. Well, unlike the writers of that piece I actually read the publications and not just the press release of a prostate cancer charity. There were in fact two studies reported together with a lengthy editorial. The first study was American and produced a negative result. The larger European study was of borderline statistical significance and for the statistically literate amongst you, showed a 20% relative risk reduction of cancer specific mortality over a 10 year period with a p value of <0.04. Never mind the stats, translated into numbers that all lay men could understand, you would need to screen 1,400 men for 10 years to save one prostate cancer death at the expense of over-diagnosing 48 cases of cancer that would be treated with radical surgery that frequently lead to impotence and incontinence and on rare occasions death from the complications of surgery. The editorial concluded that it was premature to make any kind of recommendation and urged that we waited for the outcome of the British trial. That happens to be the study I chair. I can claim no credit for the elegant and ambitious design of that trial that is all down to the three principle investigators, Freddie Hamdy, Jenny Donovan and David Neal. I was invited in as an independent chairman to see fair play. 400,000 men in the UK have been randomized to PSA screening or not. Those with a raised PSA are further investigated and if in the end their prostate biopsies showed localized cancer they are then offered re-randomization to three treatment groups, radical surgery, radical radiotherapy or "active monitoring". The two primary outcome measures are cancer specific mortality and the rate of over-diagnosis. Health economics is factored in as well and the secondary randomization will allow measures of quality of life as well as length of life in the different treatment groups, whilst the "active monitoring" arm will allow us to study the natural history of screen detected prostate cancer. This latter group will also allow us to study the molecular biology of the disease to see if we can learn to separate out the "poodles" (cancers that will remain latent for the duration of life) from the "Rottweiler's" (those that are predetermined to invade and spread). If only we had our time over again *that* is how the breast cancer trials should have been designed!

Is There a Reasonable "Exit Strategy"?

Let me summarize in a series of bullet points where we have arrived with breast cancer screening.

- The current NHS screening programme is based on the results of randomized controlled trials that were published before 1987 and started in the late 1960s and early 1970s
- Some of these trials in retrospect were of poor quality
- With mature follow up and repeated attempts at meta-analysis, the relative risk reduction (RRR) in breast cancer specific mortality has been estimated as running at about 13%-16% depending on the selection criteria of trials to be included.
- In absolute terms therefore the numbers needed to screen to prevent one breast cancer death is about 1:2,000. Anything better than this depends on mathematical manipulation of the data that I either simply don't understand or is based on those self -selected women who accept the invitation to screen. ("selection bias")
- Along the way the estimates of harm have increased. At the outset the hazards of over-diagnosis were ignored, then as the rate of screen detected duct carcinoma in situ (DCIS) shot up it was still judged to

be worth the cost. Now we recognize that the over-diagnosis of "pseudo" invasive cancers is a problem. The extent of over-diagnosis is debateable but I personally agree that if you include DCIS and IDC it mounts to about 10 cases treated unnecessarily for every life saved.

- Putting politics aside for the moment I wonder how many of us would have voted for the NHSBSP in 1987 knowing what we know today.
- Furthermore, in spite of the wonderful advances we've made in imaging technology and treatment in the last 20 years there has been only one new trial reported for screening and that was the trial for the under 50s that was essentially negative. [12]
- In other words we are using state of the art imaging and modern therapy to service a programme based on data that is 20 years old. It is also worth re-iterating at this juncture that improvements in the treatment of symptomatic patients since the mid 1980s leaves a much narrower window of opportunity for screening, so that even our estimates of1: 2,000 based on these old trials might have to be multiplied by a factor of about 0.6.

So where do we go from here? I think to close the programme is both scientifically and politically unacceptable. I therefore want to make two practical propositions for research and development. One concerns "person preferences" and the other concerns the more efficient use of scarce resources that I will refer to as risk assessment/risk management (RARM)

Person Preference

Since 1995 when I resigned from the NHSBS committee I have publically expressed my concerns on the issue of informed choice for women invited for screening. This has often led to ridicule and *ad hominum* attacks. I take no particular pleasure in the fact that the NHS has at last accepted the point and agreed to rewrite the letters of invitation.

From The Times February 21, 2009
"NHS rips up breast cancer leaflet and starts all over again"

My concern is that they will repeat the mistakes of the past if we leave this task to the usual suspects. Furthermore it's not for me to prejudge what level of benefit and what level of harm might influence the average woman to accept the invitation. For this reason I think there are two related areas of research. First the development of an information pack that includes decision aids. This could be used in a person preference study where well women might be offered sliding scales of benefits and harms to find the point at which screening is judged acceptable. These data might then inform the next and perhaps more important area of research on more efficient ways of using scarce resources in the NHS.

RARM

The beauty of a risk assessment risk management is that it provides a platform for the management of all women in an attempt to reduce the incidence as well as the mortality from breast cancer where mammographic screening is one component of an integrated programme. The first step is to set up a facility nation wide for risk assessment using one of the modern computer programmes. Women would then be *offered* not *compelled* to accept this service. Initially a practice nurse could administer this questionnaire but it would be quite easy to transfer this to a web- based programme for the computer literate members of the community. From the read-out an initial triage could be agreed. Those at the most extreme end of the risk spectrum, say with a relative risk (RR) of >10.0, could be invited to a clinical genetics consultation. At the other extreme those with a RR of say <2.0 might be reassured and given lifestyle advise on diet, alcohol and exercise. Those in between could then be invited to a special clinic for the second step. At this clinic women of 45 or older could have a mammogram to determine breast density that might also be kept as a baseline but also provide additional evidence about risk. (The greater the mammographic density the higher the risk) Those with radiological abnormality at this stage would be investigated in the accepted way. If the mammographic density is low and the repeat estimate falls below a RR of 2.0 then they would be reassured and given lifestyle advice. Those that remain with a RR 2.0-10.0 would be offered screening. In addition, those who were pre-menopausal might be offered prevention with tamoxifen and those who were post-menopausal could be offered entry into the IBIS II trial, a study comparing tamoxifen with arimidex for the chemo-prophylaxis of breast cancer). A recent paper in JNCI supports the validity of this approach. [13]

Conclusion

To carry on regardless is no longer acceptable neither is political spin the answer. Women are now getting smarter and the demand for change doesn't just come from grumpy old men like me but also from the legions of wise women represented by the signatories of the letter in the Times. However the changes I have in mind are not destructive but constructive. The NHSBSP has indirectly lead to the provision of the best specialist services for the diagnosis and treatment of symptomatic breast cancer in the world, riding on the back of the screening units. The centralization of care has led to the rapid recruitment into RCTs for the treatment of cancer that is the major contributor to the dramatic fall in breast cancer mortality in the UK over the last two decades. If we can now add to this the prevention of the disease and a risk adjusted screening programme then everyone is a winner.

References

[1] "Breast screening: the facts—or maybe not", Gøtzsche PC et al. *BMJ* 2009, 338; 446-448.

[2] Mortality results from a randomized prostate screening trial. Andriole et al. *NEJM* 2009, 360: 1310-1319.

[3] Screening and prostate cancer mortality in a randomized European trial. Schroder et al. *NEJM* 2009, 360:1320-1328.

[4] U.S. Preventive Services Task Force. Screening for Breast Cancer: Recommendations and Rationale. *Ann Intern Med* 2002;137: 344-6.

[5] *Screening and choice:* Informed choice for screening: implications for evaluation. Les Irwig, Kirsten McCaffery, Glenn Salkeld, Patrick Bossuyt: *BMJ* 2006;332:1148-1150.

[6] Rate of over-diagnosis of breast cancer 15 years after end of Malmö mammographic screening trial: follow up study. Zackrisson S, Andersson I, Manjer J and Garne JP, *BMJ* 2006;332:689-92.

[7] "Should I be tested for Cancer?" H Gilbert Welch. University of California Press, 2004, ISBN 0520239768.

[8] Incidence of breast cancer in Norway and Sweden during introduction of nationwide screening: prospective cohort study. Zahl PH, Strand BH, Maehlen J. *BMJ*. 2004 Apr 17;328(7445):921-4.

[9] "Randomised Clinical Trials: the patient`s point of view." Hazel Thornton, in Ductal Carcinoma in Situ of the Breast. Ed. Melvin Silverstein. Williams and Wilkins 1997.

[10] Insurance repercussions of mammographic screening: What do women think? Claire Davey, Victoria White, Jenette E. Ward. *Medical Science Monitor* 2003; 8:LE44-45.

[11] Effect of mammographic screening from age 40 years on breast cancer mortality at 10 years' follow up: a randomised controlled trial. Moss SM, Cuckle H, Evans A, Johns L, Waller M, Bobrow L, *The Lancet* 2006, 368; 2053-2060.

[12] Prevention of Breast Cancer in Postmenopausal Women: Approaches to Estimating and Reducing Risk: Steven R. Cummings, Jeffrey A. Tice, Scott Bauer, Warren S. Browne, Jack Cuzick et al; *J Natl Cancer Inst* 2009;101: 384 – 398.

Chapter 36

The Cancer "Tsar" Announces Independent Review of Screening for Breast Cancer

(Letter to the BMJ Oct.2011)

In November 2010, a group of 27 experts from around the world wrote a letter that was published synchronously, in the *BMJ* (BMJ 2010; 341:c6152) and the Times. In these communications we reviewed the emerging evidence that challenged the status quo about screening mammography, describing new evidence that suggested the estimates of benefit had been exaggerated and that the estimates of harm had been minimized. We described the benefits in absolute numbers rather relative risk reductions. The rather impressive relative risk reduction in breast cancer mortality that is now accepted as 15%, translates in absolute terms into 2,000 women need to be screened over 10 years in order to avoid one cause specific death. Incidentally there is no evidence so far that this then translates into a reduction of death from all causes. It is therefore somewhat misleading when the screening industry claim they are saving lives. Our leading concern about the harmful side at this time was the unequivocal evidence concerning the over-diagnosis and overtreatment of breast cancer detected at screening. By this we meant the increased detection of in-situ disease and good prognosis invasive disease without any change in the incidence of poor prognosis cases. In other words "cancers" that if left undetected would never have emerged to threaten a woman's life. Over-treatment of these indolent "pseudo-cancers" has involved surgery, radiotherapy and chemotherapy. Furthermore, contrary to all the promises of the screeners, mastectomy rates have increased in absolute terms in the population screened. It is also worth noting in passing, that one of the late consequences of radiotherapy for early breast cancer is an increase in deaths from ischaemic heart disease. Although in absolute terms this excess is modest, it could easily nullify the one in 2,000 chance of avoiding death from breast cancer.

We concluded our letter by suggesting that time was ripe for an independent review. I was therefore delighted to note that the BMJ has just published a letter from the cancer Tsar, Prof Mike Richards, announcing that an independent review will now take place. (BMJ 2011;343:d6843, doi: 10.1136/bmj.d6894) Although delighted to learn of this review, I remain deeply concerned about a number of issues raised in his response. My first concern is that the co-chairmen are to be Mike Richards himself and Harpal Kumar, chief executive of CRUK. Mike Richards is hardly independent as judged by his comments on radio, television and print newspapers on Wednesday the 26th of October, the day of the BMJ press release. The independence of the CRUK can be judged by its website from which I now quote.

> "We want targeted action to be taken to improve the numbers of people attending screening….
>
> We believe there are several important steps that the Government needs to take to ensure these are met to reduce variations in the screening programmes across the UK. In particular this involves:
>
> - Ensuring that screening services are adequately staffed to screen people at the appropriate time and provide them with their results quickly;
> - Finding new ways to encourage those who aren't taking part in screening to participate;
> - Improving the collection of information on how services are running and which people are being left out."

The next rather amusing ruling was that this independent review panel would be selected from those who have never previously expressed an opinion, or published a paper, related to screening for breast cancer. It would be rather like me being invited to adjudicate on climate change. Nevertheless I understand and to an extent sympathize with his motives for this. There is no doubt that the experts in this field are completely polarized and any attempt to achieve a consensus amongst the cognoscenti is guaranteed to fail. I am reminded of the fierce controversy concerning surgery for early breast cancer that raged in the early 1970s. A consensus panel on that occasion, of which I was a member, broke up in disarray. And I think that was the occasion when the expression "*consensus: nonsensus*", was coined. In the end it was left to clinical trials comparing radical versus conservative surgery to resolve the debate. How should one therefore respond to this polarization of opinion concerning screening amongst those who have *actually studied the subject and published in learning journals*? One could argue that the expert medical scientific community as a whole has reached the point of group equipoise. When such times occur, it is futile to attempt to arrive at a consensus, the correct, and scientific approach is to recognize that there is communal uncertainty, and then to carry out randomized controlled trials that would truly weigh in the balance the outcomes of both points of view in terms of lives and breasts saved. Prof Richards, in his letter to the BMJ describes a clinical trial that is about to start and for a moment my heart lifted at this prospect. With some difficulty I was able to track down the details of this study that can be found in the following web site. (Evaluating the net effects of extending the age range for breast screening in the NHS Breast Screening Program in England from 50 - 70 years to 47 - 73 years. http://www.controlled-trials.com/ISRCTN33292440) I was dismayed to learn that this huge and expensive trial will simply be comparing the current of screening program for women between the ages of 40 and 70, with an extended program that embraces a younger and older cohort. The trial simply does not address the dilemma we face concerning the harm versus benefit of screening at any age. I would therefore urge Prof. Richards to postpone the start of such a trial at least until we have the results of the expert Independent Review. However I have a much better idea for resolving the conflict. Why not use the existing infrastructure of the NHS breast-screening program for a risk adjusted approach to screening? We have excellent computer systems that allow us to accurately predict the risk of the individual developing breast cancer. I would suggest that using these tools we could undertake a triage. Those at the very highest risk are the very ones who would benefit from genetic counseling and genetic testing with screening reserved for those women who test positive but are reluctant to accept prophylactic mastectomy. At the other extreme, those women with a low to in intermediate risk of developing the disease who are 25 to 50 times more likely to die of diseases other than breast cancer; the most likely cause of death amongst this population would be cardiovascular disease. These women need counseling on how to avoid cardiovascular disease and it so happens the lifestyle interventions to reduce the risk of cardiovascular disease, e.g. exercise, avoiding obesity, controlling alcohol intake and eating lots of fresh fruit and vegetables, will incidentally reduce the risk of breast cancer. For those women in the middle group, for example with a risk ratio of 3-8, I suspect that mammographic screening as currently conducted will achieve a very much better profile of benefit versus harm. I would therefore like to suggest that instead of the randomized controlled trial proposed by Prof Richards, we should compare the conventional "one size fits all" approach, with a risk assessment/risk management scheme that I've just described. Furthermore we could use this platform for a secondary randomization for those women with screen detected duct carcinoma in situ that would involve active treatment versus active monitoring. This way we will learn something about the nature of these precursor lesions and learn how to predict those that are more likely to progress and those more likely to regress. Although this sounds somewhat radical this is precisely what we are doing in the ProtecT trial for screen-detected prostate cancer. In the prostate screening trial we are randomizing early prostate cancer between surgery, radiotherapy and active monitoring. As independent chairman of the International steering committee for this trial, I can assure the professional and lay public the study has been judged ethical and the majority of men recruited accepts randomization and seem to understand that this is the best way of resolving uncertainty. I therefore throw myself at the mercy of Prof Mike Richards begging him to consider this approach as a way of breaking the deadlock, accepting the nature of uncertainty, recognizing that the laudable way of dealing with uncertainty is to conduct a clinical trial addressing the main reasons for the polarization of expert opinion, and not to waste valuable resources on a trial which will provide no useful answer to the current dilemma. It is highly unlikely that one group of experts is 100% correct and another group of experts is 100% wrong: there must be a middle way.

In the meantime, *shush,* don't let our womenfolk know about this controversy otherwise it will frighten their pretty little heads, as it is a well known fact that women are incapable of absorbing complex information and reaching an informed decision!

Chapter 37

The Marmot Report: Accepting the Poisoned Chalice

(Editorial: British Journal of Cancer (2013) 108, 2198–2199)

"The pellet with the poison's in the vessel with the pestle; the chalice from the palace has the brew that is true!"

That catchy little verse came from a film I remember called *The Court Jester,* a musical comedy starring Danny Kaye and Glynis Johns that was screened in 1955. I think the members of the Marmot commission must have been alerted that the chalice from the palace (of Westminster) carried the true brew. Unlike Marmot et al (1) I chose to commit professional suicide by taking the hemlock in the manner of Socrates. (2)

On re-reading the full report on the "true brew" I'm astonished to see the level of uncertainty expressed in many sections of the report.

For example there are 9 expressions of uncertainty in the executive summary. These include estimates of the extent of over-diagnosis after 20 years of screening varying from 0% to 50% and estimates of benefits varying between 1:250 to 1:2000 breast cancer deaths avoided after 10 years of screening. They even go so far as to state, "Given the uncertainties around the estimates, the figures quoted give a spurious impression of accuracy". These wide ranges of estimates are based on calculations from equal numbers of "distinguished professors" on each side of the debate and we are not talking confidence intervals (CI) here. What we are observing is either a clash of ideologies or so much uncertainty as to suggest that the profession is in a state of perfect equipoise. If the former is true then one has to ask which side of the debate has the greatest conflict of interest, if the latter then we can only resolve the differences by launching a new set of randomized controlled trials that involve modern diagnostic techniques, state of the art of adjuvant systemic therapy and "safer" ways of delivering radiotherapy. Failing that we will forever be stuck in a time warp based on trials conducted 20-30 years ago.

I strongly advocate the recognition of uncertainty in the noble pursuit of evidence-based medicine and by way of encouraging this healthy state of mind recently published a paper in the BMJ wherein I tried my best to calculate the range of possible outcomes for breast cancer deaths avoided balanced against deaths resulting from the over-diagnosis and overtreatment of women gratuitously being subjected to surgery, radiotherapy and adjuvant systemic therapy. (3) Central to these calculations is the recognition that as systemic therapy improves, the window for the impact of screening narrows substantially, (4) and as over-diagnosis rates increase then the importance of the relatively rare lethal toxicities of treatment increase. If we accept the Marmot estimate of reduction in cause specific mortality of 20%, then, factoring in the role of adjuvant systemic therapy that was adopted in the years since the data accumulated to provide this estimate, we would now have to screen 2,500 women for 10 years to avoid one breast cancer death.

Next, considering the toxic effects of over-diagnosis, I made use of the most comprehensive examination of rates in the USA that was recently published in the New England Journal of Medicine, and appeared a few weeks after the Marmot report. (5) In this paper Bleyer and Welch estimate that about 30% of all cancers or 50% of those detected by screening are over-diagnosed each year in the United States of America. This is a similar number to that reported by the Nordic Cochrane Centre. (6) In absolute terms this means that 70,000 women each year in the USA are told that they have breast cancer, yet their pathology will not become life threatening. The UK has a fifth of the population of the US, and if the NHS breast screening programme (NHSBSP) widens its age limits to match the US, 14,000 more women a year would be exposed to the risks of treatment with no hope of benefit.

The Early Breast Cancer Trialists' Collaborative Group overview of trials involving radiation estimated a relative risk of 1.78 for deaths from lung cancer and 1.27 for deaths from myocardial infarction in the irradiated group. (7) These data were relevant when women were recruited into the old screening trials and, despite reassurances that they don't apply today, I remain concerned. The left anterior descending coronary artery is in the field of treatment and remains at risk despite recent advances. (8) It is worth noting that, according to this latest analysis, the risks of deaths from MI from radiotherapy to the breast occur in the early years, before screening can express its potential for benefit. For these reasons, any estimates of benefits and harms based on trials reported 20 to 25 years ago, as described in the Marmot report, are irrelevant to the modern practice of medicine. It is exceptionally difficult to calculate the benefit to harm ratios based on all the developments in the past 25 years since the NHSBSP started, but my crude estimate is that for every 10,000 women invited for screening, 3 to 4 breast cancer deaths are avoided but along the way about 120 to 140 cases will be over-diagnosed. Four fifths of these women would receive radiotherapy and would be at an increased risk of dying of ischemic heart disease and lung cancer. Knowing the background risks and multiplying these by the factors 1.27 and 1.78 gives us increases of 2.0% for lung cancer and 1.33% for myocardial infarction. Adding that to all cause mortality rates I crudely estimate that an additional 1 to 3 deaths might be expected from other causes for every breast cancer death avoided. (3) *Given the uncertainties around the estimates, the figures quoted might give a spurious impression of accuracy.* It is even possible that my worst estimate is too optimistic because of two papers I overlooked in the past that describe the risk of stroke following radiotherapy to the breast (9,10) and one very recent letter to the N Engl J Med on the early risk of cardiovascular deaths amongst patients with cancer, from the act of surgery alone. (11)

Finally it is worthy of comment that the remit of the Marmot commission excluded health economics and the silence on this matter is deafening.

If we consider opportunity costs and distributive justice, I can think of many better ways of spending £100,000,000 a year. I'm writing this piece on "Red Nose Day" and have just calculated that the sums of money spent on mammographic screening in the UK and USA alone could save 500,000 innocent children in Africa dying from malaria, each year. (12)

I accept that the conclusions of the Marmot committee are the first step in the right direction but not the last word on the subject and I feel sure they would agree.

References

[1] Independent UK Panel on Breast Cancer Screening. The benefits and harms of breast cancer screening: an independent review. *Lancet* 2012; 380:1778-86.

[2] May J, Baum M, Bewley S, Plato's Socratic dialogues and the epistemology of modern medicine. *J Royal Soc Med* 2010; 103: 484-489.

[3] Baum M, Harms from breast cancer screening outweigh benefits if death caused by treatment is included. *BMJ* 2013; 346: 27.

[4] Burton RC, Bell RJ, Thiagarajah G, Stevenson C. Adjuvant therapy, not mammographic screening, accounts for most of the observed breast cancer specific mortality reductions in Australian women since the national screening program began in 1991. *Breast Cancer Res Treat* 2012;131:949-55.

[5] Bleyer A, Welch HG, Effect of three decades of screening mammography on breast-cancer incidence. *N Eng J Med* 2012;367: 1998-2005.

[6] Gøtzsche PC, Nielsen M. Screening for breast cancer with mammography. *Cochrane Database Syst Rev* 2011;(1):CD001877.

[7] Clarke M, Collins R, Darby S, Davies C, Elphinstone P, Evans E, et al. Effects of radiotherapy and of differences in the extent of surgery for early breast cancer on local recurrence and 15-year survival: an overview of the randomised trials. *Lancet* 2005; 366:2087-106.

[8] Darby SC, Ewertz M, McGale P, Bennet AM, Blom-Goldman U, BrØnnum D, et al, Risk of Ischemic Heart disease in Women after Radiotherapy for Breast Cancer. *N Engl J Med* 2013; 368: 987-998.

[9] Nilsson G, Holmberg L, Garmo H, Terent A and Blomquist C. Increased incidence of stroke in women with breast cancer. *European journal of Cancer* 2005; 41: 423-429.

[10] Nilsson G, Holmberg L, Garmo H, Terent A and Blomquist C. Radiation to supraclavicular and internal mammary nodes in breast cancer increases the risk of stroke. *British Journal of Cancer* 2009; 100: 811-816.

[11] Voskoboynik M, Urban P, Mileshkin L. Early cardiovascular deaths in patients with cancer. *N.Engl J Med* 2012; 367:1572-3.

[12] http://www.rednoseday.com/whats-going-on/mary-and-martha

Chapter 38

To Screen or Not to Screen: Daily Mail

(With acknowledgments to journalist Spencer Bright's support, October 31st 2012)

For 17 years I've been saying that Britain's breast-screening programme has been over-diagnosing cases of breast cancer, forcing thousands of women to undergo unnecessary treatment that potentially can be physically disfiguring, psychologically damaging and seriously detrimental to their health. So I was delighted to see the results of the review carried out by Professor Sir Michael Marmot and his team being published and deservedly hitting the headlines with its central finding: that although the £100 million NHS programme saves 1,300 lives a year, some 4,000 women a year are undergoing unnecessary treatments that can includes lumpectomy, mastectomy and even radio therapy.

My pleasure was not born out of some selfish delight in being able to say, "I told you so" but out of the satisfaction that, for the first time, women are to be given the full facts about breast screening. Yes, it will pick up previously undetected breast tumours but because of the uncertainty in determining which tumours will prove to be almost harmless and which will be aggressively life-threatening, there is a real risk that any woman diagnosed as having a tumour will undergo unnecessary treatment.

Indeed, the risk could be even higher than that published this week. For while the Marmot review has gone public with a figure of three women being treated unnecessarily for every life saved, other estimates – and my own gut feeling borne out of a medical career dedicated to fighting this dreadful disease – is that the figure could be closer to ten-to-one.

But now is not the time to quibble over statistics; now is the time to quietly celebrate the fact that at long last women will get all the facts about breast screening, finally bringing them into line with the prostate cancer-screening program for men. There – and I speak as the independent chairman of an on-going review of the prostate screening programme – it has long been accepted that the simple blood test used for the early detection of prostate tumours (the so-called PSA test) will over-diagnose tumours and entire research programmes are dedicated to eliminating the unnecessary treatments that potentially result. The Marmot review – and the recommendation that flow from its findings – will simply provide women with the same amount of information as men.

In both cases, the screening programmes will pick up tumours. But now all patients - women and men - will be told there is a chance that a tumour may not need treatment and that there is a risk of any treatment turning out to be worse than the disease. Radiotherapy for breast cancer, for instance, a treatment that 80 per cent of all breast cancer patients receive, can cause serious and potentially life-threatening damage to the arteries of the heart that takes 10 or more years to show up. Women need to know this.

In the recent past, my publicly expressed doubts over the effectiveness of the breast-screening programme has resulted in me being labelled “a misogynist” or even “a killer of women” by my critics. But nothing could be further from the truth. My mother died of breast cancer at a relatively early age, my sister is a long-term survivor of the disease and, at present, there are 17 young women in my family at risk of developing the disease. It’s on their behalf that I’ve charged into battle against this terrible disease – first as a cancer surgeon and one time co-director of the first breast-screening programme to be introduced in this country, in London and the South East.

It took about ten years for my first doubts to set in, that we might be doing more harm than good and, when a number of research studies started to support my view, I resigned from the NHS Breast Screening committee in 1995. It is appalling that it has taken another 17 years for the NHS and its Government employers to admit what research has told them time and again - that the benefits of breast screening were being greatly exaggerated.

The problems arise from the difficulties in determining the relatively harmless breast tumours from the killers, the poodles from the Rottweiler, if you like. Some 20 per cent of the breast tumours picked up by the screening programme are so-called duct carcinomas in situ (DCIS) of which I'd estimate that less than a third will prove to be aggressive and life-threatening.

That has been well known for some time but what has been appreciated more recently is that a significant percentage of invasive breast tumours – traditionally regarded as the worst kind – won't develop in a life-threatening way either.

An entire cancer-aware generation has grown up believing that early diagnosis can only be a good thing. But when that diagnosis results in premature, debilitating, life-changing treatment then that's simply not the case. There can't be a surgeon in the world who would want to perform an unnecessary mastectomy, just as no radiotherapist would want to risk damaging a patient's heart (the heart lying directly below the breast) in the process of killing a tumour that actually poses little or no threat.

The problem is the diagnostic uncertainty. Sometimes a biopsy will tell you exactly what sort of tumour you are dealing with but sometimes it won't. Reducing this uncertainty requires more research but until now this sort of research has been hampered by the accepted NHS wisdom that breast screening was, by definition, a good thing. Women couldn't possibly be asked to opt out of something that might well save their life was the official line.

Well, thanks to the Marmot review and its admission that screening – and the treatments that result – could very well be injurious to life, women may well be interested in taking part in such research projects, just as men have been for similar research to improve then diagnosis of prostate cancer.

Should the NHS abandon its breast-screening programme in the wake of the Marmot findings? Certainly not, the knowledge and expertise built up over the past quarter of a century is far too valuable for that to be a sensible option. But it does need to be better targeted.

Some 5 per cent of women, courtesy of a ghastly genetic inheritance, are at such high risk of developing breast cancer that they need to be taken out of the routine screening programme altogether to be treated by specialists in genetic diseases instead.

It's my belief that the 70 per cent of women at low-risk of developing breast cancer should also be taken out of the screening programme, with the money saved being spent on an approach that treats the health of the woman as a whole rather than one specific disease. They need to be educated about the risk, prevention and early detection of cardio-vascular disease (which kills five times as many women as breast cancer) lung cancer, ovarian cancer, osteoporosis, and of course, breast cancer.

But it's the 25 per cent of women at medium-to-high risk of developing breast cancer who are likely to benefit most from staying in a regular screening programme and there are well-established statistical formula for establishing who they are. Women with one or more close relatives who have had breast cancer; women who had their children over the age of thirty; women who began their periods early; women who entered the menopause late; women who drink over the safe limits of alcohol – all these women would have good reason for staying in a programme of regular mammograms.

But, thanks to the Marmot review, those women will know what their mothers, aunts and older sisters were never told – that there is a risk of over-diagnosis and that some treatments may be unnecessary and damaging to their health.

But they can also take comfort from one more thing, which hasn't changed. If the worst happens and a life-threatening breast cancer is diagnosed, they'll get the best possible treatment that modern medical science can offer and that in itself has led to the dramatic 40% drop in mortality in the last 20 years even for the younger women who were never screened. After all, isn't that what a good healthcare system should be all about – the latest research, the fullest possible information for patients and the best treatments available? And, at long last, with breast cancer, we finally seem to be getting there.

Chapter 39

Breaking News

This subject moves on so quickly with hardly a week passing by without another nail hammered into the coffin of the screening cadaver and yet the zombie continues to prey upon its victims! Two recent examples come to mind. The 25-year follow up of the National Canadian trial, one of the few with robust methodology, was recently published in the British Medical Journal. [1] The outcomes for breast cancer mortality and overall mortality remained superimposed throughout this long period of follow up.

The second remarkable publication I wish to draw to your attention to, is the conclusions of the Swiss Medical Board published in the prestigious New England Journal of Medicine. [2] They can claim the credit to be first nation to advocate the dismantling of their national screening program.

References

[1] Twenty-Five year follow up for breast cancer incidence and mortality of the Canadian National Breast Screening study: randomised screening trial. *BMJ* 348; g 366, 2014 (February 11th)

[2] Abolishing Mammography Screening programs? A view from the Swiss Medical Board. Biller-Adorno N and Jüni P, April 16th 2014

Towards Synthesis

A miscellany of ephemera and essays that demonstrate how the life of a sceptic not only encourages scientific discovery, but can also fuel a healthy attitude to life in general and also provide a meaning to this *brief candle*

Chapter 40

"2084" A Play in Three Acts (With Acknowledgments to George Orwell)

First performed and the European Breast Cancer Conference (EBCC)
Barcelona 2004

Act 1

Narrator (in a deep portentous voice): The year is 2084, the 70th anniversary of the foundation of the United States of Europe (USE). For the last 70 years the Politically Correct party have been in power; a rainbow alliance of the Post Modern Party, the Organic Green Party, Euro-American Tobacco Company (EAT) and the Animal Liberation Front (ALF).

The European Federation of States came about after the cataclysmic events of 2011-2014. The Euro, the then currency of the Eurozone was facing collapse because the Italian and Greek governments had forgotten to collect tax for about 5 years and most European citizens were taking their State pensions at the age of 50. In order to save the Euro, the French and German leaders, President Nicholas Sarkozy and Chancellor Angela Merkle, decided on plans for fiscal union across the zone. David Cameron, prime minister of what was then known as the United Kingdom, broke ranks and tried to go it alone. The Eurozone then reacted by erecting huge tariff barriers for trade thus leading to the collapse of the British economy. The UK had no other choice but to join the Eurozone. Fiscal union was then followed by a number of draconian acts in the European parliament by unelected technocrats, that led to a full Federal union of states with, for example common defense, science and education policies. In spite of all this the Euro collapsed and was replaced with the Deutchefrank (DF). The DF was kept afloat by selling bonds to the Chinese. By 2064 the world was divided into three warring financial markets. The dollar collapsed in 2055 when the health care budget reached 115% of the GDP and the USA was forced to join the United States of North and South America, now known as the Pesozone. The third major power was the Yuan zone that included China, Russia, Japan and the rest of the world. It was founded in 2050 when oil reserves in the Middle East ran out and fossil fuel was all that was left. To their credit the Yuan zone was the only part of the world that actually manufactured anything. Global warming increased as a result but stabilized once the global population had shrunk by 3 billion. China proudly contributed to this fall in global population by abandoning westernized medicine in favour of Traditional Chinese Medicine (TCM). Sub Sahara Africa is now an arid unpopulated desert and the rhinoceros has been extinct for 30 years. Initially this was a problem for TCM in the management of impotence but with typical Chinese ingenuity powdered rhinoceros horn has been replaced by cucumber sandwiches. Talking of which, the summer of 2084 in London has been glorious continuing its sub-tropical climate of recent years.

The curtain rises in the office of the Governor of England, a minor off shore state close to the European mainland. The Governor, Ranjit Karma Sutra, is seated at his desk. Behind his desk is a flag bearing the red cross of St George, a rather pathetic vestige from the days when England had a decent football team. Standing in front of the desk is the state director of the Ministry of Truth and Health, Humphrey Steadfast, and the cancer Tsar, Professor Cliff Richards. They all wear Bermuda shorts and Hawaiian shirts.

Scene 1

Governor: What's the excitement Humphrey? You look as if you ran up the stairs, the two of you. Not another damn Federal health initiative I hope?

Steadfast: No sir, this time it's good news. We've cracked the problem of Federal directive; screening, 2083 number 12A subsection little iii.

Governor: Remind me what that is Humphrey. I can't keep up with this never-ending flood of health directives from Brussels.

Steadfast: It's the one about comprehensive screening for all cancers from the cradle to the grave. The cradle bit is my silly attempt at irony; in fact it's not meant to start until they attend kindergarten. You said it was going to be impossible and cost every DF we've allocated to our health budget. Well you're half right about the cost but it's not impossible and my working party headed up by Cliff Richard here, our cancer Tsar, has cracked the problem and I've come up with an ingenious plan for covering the expense I'll get Cliff to explain the science and then I'll explain the economics.

Cliff Richards: Well Sir our breakthrough in thinking was to replace 6 different screening modalities for breast, cervix, prostate, colon, lung and ovary, by one whole body scan. This would also be supplemented by transferring half the responsibility into the hands of the lay public, literally, by making monthly self-examinations mandatory. They would of course include BSE, TSE, PRE and PSE.

G. Don't you mean PSA?

CR. No Sir, PSE stands for prostate self examination (G. nodes and grunts sagely) Coming back to the whole body scan, we set up a pilot scheme in Chelsea based at the Federal Marsden Hospital, to evaluate the Siemen's whole body virtual reality holographic endo-metabolic view engine. We call it SEIVE for short..

Governor (interrupting): What's this got to do with semen? I thought we were talking about cancer not in vivo fertilization.

Cliff: Sorry Sir. Seimens is the manufacturer based in Munich in the Federal state of Germany and they make the machine. The principle behind it is to measure and image the points of anaerobic metabolism with the subject at rest and then translate that into a free floating three dimensional holographic image than can be manoeuvred in virtual reality to inspect every nook and cranny of the human body with a resolution of 100 microns that is equivalent to about 10 cells. We then inject radioisotope labelled metabolites specific to the organ of suspicion to confirm the malignant nature of the cells. Our pilot study has demonstrated 100% sensitivity.

Governor: Hang on a moment, if I remember correctly you have to wait some time before you can be sure you've captured all the disease before you can be sure of the sensitivity. Don't you have the odd case of cancer presenting between scans?

Cliff: Excellent point sir, exactly. The fact we know we have 100% sensitivity is that 100% of our 1,000 volunteers have scanned positive!

Governor: Goodness gracious me! 100%! That means we catch all these early cancers, treat them early and effectively prevent the disease ever materializing. Congratulations gentlemen. Won't it be very expensive to detect all these early cancers and then treat them?

Steadfast: First of all sir, it would be political suicide not to implement these plans. Next think of the money we might save in avoiding all those late cancers. Yes it will be expensive: in fact my estimate is exactly as you predicted, that the cost would exceed the total annual budget for our beloved Federal Health Service. It is at this point I want to explain how it will be cost neutral. You look sceptical but you may have forgotten two advantages of our Federal status. Firstly by the statute of creative accountancy 2079, section 23, we are allowed to offset the opportunity costs in a top down trans-allocation every 6 months between the purchasing and providing wings of the FHS in each financial year. Secondly the mandatory teaching of the French Impressionist school of post-modern scientific method and arising out of that federal educational directive, 1008 iii, 2076, concerning the curriculum at the Federal homeopathic school of medicine. French post-modernism accepts any worldview on the nature of evidence. Good historic anecdotal evidence and provings for homeopathic remedies is adequate to justify its use in all diseases. As these remedies contain only the memory of a molecule of the active compound then our pharmacopoeia becomes very cheap. In fact it comes at the price of tap water that shaken not stirred, with a drop or two on a sugar pill. **[Steadfast breaks into song, "a spoonful of sugar makes the medicine go down....etc." until cautioned by Mr. Karma Sutra]** Sorry Mr. Governor, I got rather carried away there. So as I was saying, annual whole body scanning, monthly self examination, homeopathy for the cancers detected, blame it on the patient if anything goes wrong and all cost neutral!

G. Well done old boy. Well done both of you. In fact if good old King William III, were still on the throne I'd recommend both of you for a knighthood. The sound of Sir Humphrey rolls nicely off the tongue. Sadly it will have to be *legion d'honneur* first class for the two of you.

Humphrey and Cliff in unison. Thank you sir! We don't deserve it.

Scene 2

Narrator: A year has passed and the legislation, FHS/ screening/ subsections i/ii/iii have now been passed by the English State government. We are in Chelsea close to the centre of London in a laboratory at the famous Republican Marsden Hospital. The time is 0700. Slumped at his desk, his curly head in his hands; we encounter Professor Winston Smith, director of the

Dept. of Medical Oncology. He has clearly been working all night, his table strewn with paper. Cardboard cups and organic tobacco smoking tubes litter his desk. His PC flickers balefully, as a pale and damp dawn light catches the holographic sign above his door.

"THESE LABORATORIES WERE SPONSORED BY THE PC ORGANIC TOBACCO COMPANY OF EUROPE".

He wakes with a start.

Winston: Oh my G*D its 0700 already, I've been working all night and I've only got two days to go before the site visit by the USE thought police and still I haven't worked out an acceptable research program that will satisfy the Institute Director, not to mention The Party. I need help, but who can I turn to and who can I trust? These days you never know who might be employed by Federal GCP monitoring authority. (Thinks) I know! I'll get Martine Kwik-Fix, I'm sure she can be trusted. After all she has been my data manager for nearly 20 years and our affair must surely have been forgotten by now. [Picks up mobile phone and dials a number] Hello-Oh could I speak to Martine please this is urgent-me? Sorry I'm Winston Smith. [A moment passes whilst Winston lights up another tube]

Hi Martine-who answered the phone? [pause]

Oh, glad to learn that it was a state sponsored visit.

Can you please come round ASAP as I'm getting nowhere with the site visit proposals for the next quinquennial grant application. I need your sensible advice. I've been up all night and my desk is littered with cardboard cups and organic tobacco smoking tubes. [Pause] Gee thanks darling- no, come just as you are.

[Pause whilst Winston turns to his computer, pours coffee into a cup and continues to smoke]

Martine [rushing in breathless with a dressing gown thrown over her night clothes, her hair dishevelled, bust line bulging ominously carrying an empty box in her hand]

I came as quick as I could but they searched me at the entrance for non-PC materials, fortunately I had the foresight to hide the nude mice!

Loud Voice over public address system: Achtung, attention! This alert is to remind you to carry out your monthly self-examination. Failure to do will be met with a fine of 1,000 DF. We are watching you!

Martine and Winston in unison: [Jumping with surprise] Oh my gawd, oh my gawd! [Winston then turns his back on Martine and rummages in the front of his jeans. He then slips a hand down the back of his pants and struggles to perform a rectal and prostate examination himself. Martine turns her back on Winston and slips her hands down her bra retrieving them with a scream showing a mouse in each hand.]

Winston: I hate those sessions. What on earth have you got in your hands? (Inspects mice) Why on earth did you need ***to smuggle*** in the nude mice?

Martine: Don't you remember European directive 84/12,018 subsection 21A?

"All rodent experiments have been banned by the Animal Liberation Front and all naked mice must be clothed unless there is explicit consent through a murine interpreter and the experiments will benefit mice in the future."

Winston: Oh damn it! I'd forgotten that directive-there goes the first set of proposals! [Tears up sheet of paper] What about the tissue culture work using the MCF 7 cell lines and the carcinogenic effect of coal tars?

Martine: What's the matter with you Winston? Don't you remember the directive from 5 years ago enshrined in the last Declaration of Brussels? I can almost quote from memory. H'mm-Subsection 18b) "The use of any cell line for cancer research that is of human origin and where the original cell donor did not expressly condone experiments to which prospective consent had been given, is forbidden. Breach of this regulation will lead to immediate suspension."

And then of course there was the Treaty of Strasbourg at the establishment of the PC party which cemented the relationship between the Post Modern Party and E.A.T., containing a statement to the effect that any epidemiological research from the past that linked smoking to lung cancer was fundamentally flawed and only research that demonstrated the health benefits of tobacco consumption was to be funded. This was later modified to include a clause to satisfy the Organic Green Party that the tobacco must be organically grown.

Winston: [tears up second sheet of paper]

Ah well that still leaves my proposals for the study of archival material from the last ever RCT in breast cancer EORTC SELECTRON beta 2034. The new electron spin assay on the codones for the ER delta binding domains of the DNA of the oestrogen response elements on 17Q look very promising and might at least explain that paradoxical result of the ATAC trial reported 80 years ago.

Martine: But Winston I think your forgetting something. The authors of that trial never got prospective consent for this test to be used on archival patient's material.

Winston: How could they? The assay was only described two years ago!

Martine: But that's not the point, you should know by now that all biological studies on any materials taken from patients in clinical trials for one purpose cannot be used for another purpose without the patient's fully informed consent.

Winston: But that's absurd, all those patients will have died decades ago. Am I to get consent posthumously? [Laughs ironically]

Martine: Well actually you're wrong on both counts. For a start many of those patients are still alive because of the chance finding that aromatase inhibitors also inhibit telomerase activity in normal tissue. Secondly, posthumous consent is possible these days through the European Ministry of Spiritualism providing you approach a State Registered medium.

Winston: Oh come off it Martine- you don't believe all that hocus-pocus stuff do you?

Martine: SHUSH WINSTON! Don't you know the thought police of the PC Party might be bugging these labs.

Winston: Oh my gosh Martine you're right, perhaps we should continue this conversation with all the centrifuges spinning. Anyway, have you had a chance to read my proposals for a new BIG trial of the antibody raised against the molecular memory of the neonatal viral infection that causes breast cancer in mice? Thank G*D that was a natural observation that also improved the husbandry of those [raises voice a little] POOR UNFORTUNATE CREATURES OF GOD'S CREATION.

Martine: Yes the science is good but you'll never get it past the Institutional Research Ethics Committee, the MREC, the F.S.E. Research Integrity Board and the Global Ethical Imperialism Inquisition. Firstly the use of a placebo, even if it's in addition to best available therapy is forbidden under the 2067 revision of the Helsinki Declaration. Secondly, the Ministry for Alternative Medicine insists that any trial of allopathic medicine for cancer must include Iscador in all of the treatment arms. And finally, your budget calculations underestimate by about 1,000% the costs of GCP.

Winston: [losing his temper] Oh sod GCP let the F.S.E. pay for that!

[Pauses-scratches his head and eyes light up]

Mind you you've given me an idea how we can circumvent all these restrictions. Firstly, let's use Iscador 30C in all four arms of the trial as it contains the memory of water, (Ironic laugh) and is a perfect control for the molecular memory of viral antigens. Secondly, if you remember, the Ministry for Alternative Medicine has an unspent research budget of 6 billion DFs, enough to pay for 5 years of GCP. We can sell it to them as research into alternative medicine in which case it doesn't have to leap any hurdles or pass any ethical reviews.

Martine: You're brilliant Winston-of course that's the answer. This could be the first RCT launched in 70 years.

Sudden booming voice from off-stage;

That's what you think sucker!

[Crash of breaking glass, three men in balaclavas and para-military uniforms burst in and pinion Winston and Martine's arms to their sides]

Off-stage Voice:

[Singing in a childish voice- to the tune of Oranges and Lemons]

"Oranges and Lemons
James Lind's famous trial,
Your words were recorded,
Refute all denial.
It's no good resisting,
You're quite underpowered.
[In slow basso profundo]
What chance you'll survive,
Ps less than point 5 !"

Act II

Scene 1

Narrator: Three months later- the scene is the tribunal room of the Ministry of Truth and Health, MYTH for short, in Whitehall. Six sinister figures in pointed hoods with slit like eyeholes are sitting at a long table a single chair facing them. They are scanning documents and making notes. After a few moments the chairman of the tribunal, Humphrey Steadfast, throws back his hood and speaks out.

Humphrey Steadfast; Bring in the accused, Professor Winston Smith!

[Winston in bloodstained rags; a bandage round his head, his hands manacled is dragged in by the paramilitary guards and thrown on his knees by the vacant chair]

Steadfast: [In sweet tone] Please Professor Smith get off your knees and sit down. Would you like a glass of water? [Winston shakes his head and sits down]

Are you aware of the gravity of the charges against you Professor Smith?

Winston: I suppose it's to do with not getting the papers ready in time for the site visit.

Chairman: Oh no, it's much more serious than that. You are accused of not being politically correct: A crime with a penalty worse than death.

Winston: Oh no! Please not that!

Steadfast: I'm now going to hand you over to my colleagues on the tribunal who represent each of the constituencies of the Ministry of Truth and Health.

Please start the cross examination, representative of the Animal Liberation Front, A.L.F.

ALF: Please call me Alf. [With sudden passion]. When did you stop torturing defenceless little animals?

Winston: [With indignation] I've never tortured animals.

ALF: But we overheard you threatening to carry out experiments on nude mice.

Winston: But that's experimentation not torture, and in any case our mice are well cared for, better than in nature and they don't suffer any pain.

ALF: Come, come, Prof. Smith. Nothing is better than nature and how would you like to be stripped naked and have subcutaneous inoculations of cancer?

Winston: But I'm a human!

ALF: Ah Hah! The worst case of specism I've ever heard- condemned out of his own mouth. Back to you chair.

Steadfast: Over to you Madam Organic Green Party.

Madam ORG: [Sweetly] Oh please call me Orgy. We overhead you threatening to do research on the carcinogenic properties of organic tobacco, why would you wish to break the law on that?

Winston; Well as you ask, ever since that legislation was passed I've noticed an increasing incidence of lung cancer. So I just put two and two together.

Madam ORG: [screeching] -And made six! You foolish man. Don't you read the adverts? Why do you think Marlboro Man is so fit and tanned? It's because he smokes organic tobacco. Our partners from EAT have assured us on that. Further- more coughing in the morning clears the lungs. What do you think Mr. EAT?

Mr EAT: Absolutely true. In any case all this nonsense was exposed 50 years ago. The only support for the lung cancer theory was statistics. And you know what we think of statistics: lies, damn lies and statistics? [All but Winston fall about laughing]

Madam ORG: Worse than that there were even experiments on little furry rabbits forcing them to smoke! [Starts sobbing]

Mr ALF: Oh my God, I'd forgotten that. The ultimate cruelty. I suppose that kind of experimentation is not torture Professor Smith?

Winston: I've never condoned those types of experiments and what's wrong with statistics? [The tribunal collapses in laughter again]

Steadfast; [barely controlling himself holds up both hands and starts counting his fingers on his left hand] 10,9,8,7,6 plus 5 on my right hand, so I've got 11 fingers eh, Professor Winston? You can prove whatever you like with statistics.

Mr. EAT: In any case your Institution has built its labs with E.A.T. grants. Talk about biting the hand that feeds him. You are in breach of our contract with the Federal Marsden Hospital.

Madam ORG: And another thing-we overheard you daring to suggest that Iscador was only a placebo. Have you forgotten that the Party officially approves it? Even the last but one monarch of the United Kingdom, the late King Charles the III, granted the Royal Seal of approval. [Winston hangs his head]

And you were guilty of deception in trying to win financial support from the Ministry of Alternative Medicine.

Steadfast: I would like to take over the cross-examination now if you please. Prof. Smith, am I right in assuming you're against Good Clinical Practice?

Winston: That's not true, I take pride in the fact that I'm a good clinician with respect for the patients, sorry, clients. I also like to practice evidence-based medicine, oops!

Steadfast: There you go again, condemned out of your own mouth. EBM is officially unethical and forbidden by the Helsinki Declaration and the U.S.E.

Furthermore you contradict yourself, we overhead you say, [looks at notes] and I quote "Sod GCP".

Winston: Yes but that's GCP whereas I'm IN favour of good clinical practice!

Chairman: Are you mad as well as bad? [In triumph] GCP **stands** for good clinical practice! I think we've heard enough.

Cliff Richard: (Throws off hood to reveal his face whilst Winston gasps with shock.)

Wait there's worse to come! Good to see you again Winston. (Sinister laugh) I bet you thought you'd seen the last of me. Ladies and gentlemen of the tribunal, Professor Smith and I go back a long way. About 15 years ago we were both aspiring young PhD students at the European Institute of oncology in Milan. I was carrying out my seminal research on the Seimen prototype for whole body screening whilst Smith was wasting his time in the futile pursuit of a cure for cancer. He accused me and my supervisor of being in the pocket of industry and claimed that our work in trying to find earlier and earlier stages of cancer would only increase the over-diagnosis rate. Not only was it a libel it was also blasphemous in challenging a fundamental principle of faith of the Seimen's Federal European Institute of cancer. If I may quote from the second of the ten commandments of our European code of cancer research: "Thou shalt strive to catch it early, that thou mayest live forever". Once you were found guilty of that charge you were sent into internal exile in the remote gulag of the Federal Marsden Hospital hoping that you would repent on learning the error of your ways. But no, you have continued to circulate *samizdat* from your secret Facebook source continuing to claim that we are over-diagnosing cancer. Furthermore we have been monitoring your behaviour on self -examination and several times this year you have defaulted on prostate self -examination.

Winston: (in tears) But I've got a bad back!

Cliff: That's no excuse. If you apply through the appropriate channels you know very well we can send a clinical nurse specialist round to examine your prostate and complete a rectal examination for free. (Turns to Steadfast) I've nothing more to say Mr. Chairman and recommend the ultimate penalty.

[The tribunal gets into a huddle- murmuring amongst themselves for a while, before the chairman raises his head]

Steadfast: Professor Smith you are found guilty on all accounts and are condemned to Room 101.

Winston: Oh my God. What's in room 101?

Steadfast: [In sinister tone] Oh you know Professor Smith, you know- It's different for all of us, yet the same. Room 101 contains the worst of your nightmares and it goes on and on until you beg to be released from your mortal coil!

(Winston collapses and is dragged away screaming)

[Crash of drums cymbals and sudden darkness]

Scene 2

Narrator: The scene shifts to what appears to be a normal Federal Health Service clinic. Prof. Smith sits at his desk in the consultation room. He wears a white coat but looks haggard, ill at ease and twitchy. (Note to make up-white face, blue lips and dark red rings under eyes)

Winston: Next client please. [Mrs. Webwright enters: she is smartly dressed, spectacles on her forehead, high heels, clutching a huge wad of PC printout – Winston stands and holds out his hand which is ignored in an insolent manner]

Please to see you again Mrs. Webwright- [clears throat]-we now have all your results from the SEIVE test and I'm afraid the tests confirm bilateral multi-focal early breast cancer [hastens on as patient attempts to intervene] But the good news is that the tumors have the most favorable oncotype profiles and are node negative.

Mrs. W. That's not good enough Professor Smith. I want to know they are node negative on proteiomic-immunohistochemistry and if so what mono-clonal antibody was used and whether your lab is involved in the European quality control program.

[Winston tries to intervene but patient drones on in an unstoppable manner]

Furthermore it is just not good enough to claim that the oncotype is favourable. Have you tested the tumour with the new electron spin assay on the codones for the ER delta binding domains of the DNA of the oestrogen response elements on 17Q? That's essential as I may be eligible for treatment with that new molecular mimicry technique which is available at the Cancer theme park in Milan.

[Winston again tries to intervene but the flood of techno-babble is unstoppable]

I've also read reports on the remarkable clinical outcome of a patient with advanced, doxirubicin-resistant breast cancer who was later treated with DNA damaging agents, on the basis of the observation of significant activity of this class of drugs against a personalized xenograft generated from the patient's surgically resected tumor. Mitomycin C treatment, selected on the basis of its robust preclinical activity in a personalized xenograft generated from the patient's tumor, resulted in long-lasting tumor response. Global genomic sequencing revealed biallelic inactivation of the gene encoding PalB2 protein in this patient's cancer; the mutation is predicted to disrupt BRCA1 and BRCA2 interactions critical to DNA double-strand break repair. This work suggests that inactivation of the PALB2 gene is a determinant of response to DNA damage in breast cancer and a new target for personalizing cancer treatment. Integrating personalized xenografts with unbiased exomic sequencing should lead you to customized therapy, tailored to my genetic environment. Furthermore MicroRNA-155 (miR-155) is overexpressed in many breast cancers; I've read recent reports that the tumor suppressor gene suppressor of cytokine signaling 1 is an evolutionarily conserved target of miR-155 in breast cancer cells. Mir-155 expression is inversely correlated with socs1 expression in breast cancer cell lines as well as in a subset of primary breast tumors. In addition 24A-->G mutation in the miR-155 binding site of the SOCS1 3' untranslated region in a breast tumor that reduced miR-155 repression, implicating a mechanism for miRNA targets to avoid repression. I want you to look for over-expression of miR-155 in my breast cancer xenograft as it leads to constitutive activation of signal transducer and activator of transcription 3 (STAT3) through the Janus-activated kinase (JAK) pathway, and stimulation of breast cancer cells by the inflammatory cytokines IFN-gamma and interleukin-6 (IL-6), lipopolysaccharide (LPS), and polyriboinosinic:polyribocytidylic acid and significantly upregulates mir-155 expression, suggesting that miR-155 may serve as a bridge between inflammation and cancer. Taken together, all this suggests is that miR-155 is an oncomiR in breast cancer and that miR-155 may be a potential target in breast cancer therapy. So I demand personalized treatment based on my xenograft responses. Don't you agree?

Winston: Well actually no, you see ……..

Mrs.W.; ***What I*** see Professor is that you are out of date and out of touch. Call yourself a professor!? I demand a second opinion.

Winston: [Bowed and humbled] OK Mrs Webwright I'll see to that right away. Who would you like to see?

Mrs. W: [Consulting her notes] Err, Prof' Buzz Lightyear at the European Cancer Centre please and I expect the Federal Health Service to pay all my expenses. [Flounces out]

Winston: [Shakes his head sadly and takes a gulp of coffee] Next client please.

[In walks Mrs. Wholemeal- She is dressed in a long caftan and wears sandals on her feet. Her hair is long and unkempt. She wears huge chunky rings on fingers, dozens of bangles on her arms and great loops on her ears. Most noticeable is the large crystal she wears round her neck. She carries a plastic bottle of water in one hand from which she is drinking whilst smoking a cigarette in the other hand- Winston is about to say something but she puts a finger to her lips and starts chanting a mantra whilst walking three times round his chair scattering water as she goes. She looks around with a complacent smile and plumps herself down on the chair and looks expectantly at Winston]

Winstone: Well Mrs. Wholemeal we've got the results of your SEIVE scan now and I'm afraid they show suspicion of cancer in the thyroid, ovary and left adrenal gland. Fortunately they are all very early.

Mrs. W: [chortles in a good natured if patronizing way] my dear professor, how old fashioned you are. Still adhering to that ghastly allopathic classification of disease?

Now come my good man, I know I have an imbalance of my vital forces and I suspect that my Ying is out of synchrony with my Yang. Don't talk to me about multiple different cancers. I'm a whole person you know not a series of organs. In fact I find your aura rather unsympathetic. Tell me, are you a Scorpio? I'm a Virgo you know, check my notes if you don't believe it. Also the Ministry of Alternative Medicine has decreed that all patients have the right to be treated by a doctor with the astrological birth sign of their choice. I bet you're Gemini, no don't tell me I'll guess. In the meantime I want my whole-body spectral scan before I accept any treatment. Also my serum selenium, rare elements and molecular memory of mistletoe need to be measured. [Winston tries to intervene] Shush my good man. I also want referral to the hospital herbalist, homoeopathist, acupuncturist, iridologist and Ayruvedic counsellor.

[Winston starts demonstrating impatience]

Oh now I'm getting upset by your body language-feel my pulses. [Winston takes wrist]

NOT THERE stupid man, the eight pulses of my umbilicus.

Anyway I don't believe in cancer, it's just your way of medicalizing natural imbalances of nature's vital forces. And then what do you do? Earn huge sums cutting, burning and poisoning us poor people. Thank God the government had the wisdom to appoint a minister of alternative and holistic medicine and isn't Mr. Charles Windsor the spitting image of his grandfather?

Winston: Clearly Mrs. Wholemeal I'm not up to your demanding standards. I think I better refer you to the hospital's department of alternative and holistic medicine.

[Bends forward to write a note, burns it in an ashtray and makes an incantation over the smoke.]

Mrs.W; Thank you doctor. [Retreats from office after three turns round her chair sprinkling water]

Winston: Next client please!

[Enter Mr. Knowmyrights in the company of a man in a dark suit bearing a clipboard and a hand held recording device; they both sit down stony faced staring at Winston]

Good day Mr. Knowmyrights and who is your friend.

Mr. Knowmyrights: This is my medico-legal rights consultant and he will be making a recording of our consultation.

Winston: But Mr. Knowmyrights you can't have any medico-legal problems already, we've only just met.

KMR: I have, you kept me waiting five minutes and I don't like your attitude. Make a note of that will you Blomfield.

Winston: (Cowed and buckling under the strain) I'm truly sorry Sir, it won't happen again. Can I learn why you have come to consult me?

KMR: (shouting) What, you don't know already? Didn't you read the bloody letter from my bloody GP?

Winston: (Finally showing some of his metal) There's no need to shout and there's no need to use foul language. No I didn't get a bloody letter from your bloody GP, so why don't you bloody well tell me yourself why you've bloody well come to waste my time!

KMR: (Shocked into silence for a moment and mouthing like a fish) .....Did you hear that Blomfield? Did you hear how that wretch spoke to me? I hope you bloody well got it recorded. We'll report him to the Chief of the Federal Complaints Commission this very day and he'll be suspended before nightfall, and if I have my way, sentenced to life in room 101.

Winston: (jumps to his feet and starts wrestling them both out) You fools, you idiots, this is my room 101 and nothing can make it worse for me.

[Enter Mrs. Webwright and Mrs. Wholemeal together claiming they had forgotten some important questions- they speak mumbo jumbo in pseudoscientific or new age terms louder and louder, working themselves up into a frenzy of screeching. KMR and Blomfield turn around and join in the clamour]

Winston: I can't take any more of this, I can't go on –I must end it now! [Takes gun from draw]

Flash-Bang-Darkness

THE END

Chapter 41

My Thoughts on the Fifth Anniversary of 9/11

(July 2005, Unpublished)

Last night my wife and I, together with a number of our family, attended the "Last night at the Proms" at Kenwood open-air concert, Hampstead Heath. This is a delightful annual event that marks the end of the summer season. Traditionally the last few orchestral pieces include Thomas Arne's Rule Britannia, Hubert Parry's hymn "Jerusalem", using the words of William Blake's poem, and as a grand finale, Edward Elgar's Pomp and Circumstance March No.1. This is always accompanied by much waving of the Union flags by the audience and a spectacular firework display. At this point my eyes were on the audience sitting amongst the wreckage of their picnics on a grassy incline that extended as far as the eye could see. They were of all ages, all social classes and all ethnic groups. This display of jingoism was enjoyed by all as an act in self-deprecating irony that the British do so well. No one really believes that Britain rules the waves anymore but we are now much better at waiving the rules.

As I looked around I considered the charge laid against our society, as being decadent. If this is decadence then I'm all for it! I love my country and thank it for the way it treated my grandparents 100 years ago after their escape from the pogroms in Russia. I see other ethnic groups of more recent waves of immigration also having learnt to sport the union flag with that truly British touch of irony, who also have much to thank for our "imperfect" liberal democracy.

As a Boeing 747 flew peacefully overhead in a clear starlit sky, I was cruelly reminded of the events of 9/11 five years ago. To me this was a declaration of a global war against liberal democracies throughout the whole world. I am also reminded of the contribution the USA made in sacrificing tens of thousands of young men so that Europe would remain free of Nazism. If that had failed my family would have become toast. I'm reminded how the USA faced down Communism and freed Eastern Europe from its grip. Now just as we thought that was an end to history, we face a new evil ideology: Islamic fundamentalism. The destruction of the twin towers should have been the clarion call to all the free world that another threat to our freedom has emerged, with the utopian vision of a Caliphate to subjugate the world in the name of Islam. The UN wrings its hands and somehow the West, the victims, becomes the subject for vilification by an unholy alliance of the extreme left and Islamofascism.

It is my belief that our future lies in the hands of the western liberal democracies that must have the courage to believe in its values, NOT with the UN whose membership includes nations ruled by despots or kleptocrats, each enjoying equal voting rights. My evening at Kenwood was a tiny vignette of what we are defending with the genius of the composers emerging out of the age of enlightenment, describing our transition from subjugated serfs to free spirits. The most moving orchestral piece last night was the City of London's Sinfonia's passionate performance, of Smetana's Má Vlast. In this, Smetana describes the beauty of his homeland and the Czech national heritage. The central theme is a hymn to hope. That hope saw the Czech people through to the velvet revolution of the Prague Spring. My hope is that western liberal values will equip us to see off this new evil ideology of death worship in favour of the celebration of life. And YES, in partnership with our less than perfect ally the United States of America. Remember, the pursuit of perfection is the enemy of the good.

Chapter 42

Pre-Implantation Genetic Diagnosis (PGD): The Spectre of *Eugenics* or a "No Brainer"

(Editorial, International Journal Surgery. 2006;4(3):144-5.)

On Wednesday the 10th of May, the British Human Fertilisation and Embryology Authority (HFEA) gave the go ahead for pre-implantation genetic diagnosis for the selection of embryos free of the mutations that predispose to breast or colo-rectal cancer. The hysterical over reaction of some sections of the press and the television studios was predictable. On the one hand we had the shrill warnings that this was the slippery slope to "Eugenics" and on the other hand we had members of affected families saying that the decision was a "no brainer". Let me deal first of all with this reaction quickly before getting bogged down in what is a very complex ethical biomedical debate.

The tiresome morsel of American jargon, "no brainer", has slipped into common English usage quite recently and appears to have been adopted by those who have no valid opinions of their own. I suppose it stands in for "that which is self- evident", amongst English speaking people. I heard it used in a television interview with a woman in her early forties, carrying a BRCA1 mutation, a member of an extended family with a strong family history of breast and ovarian cancer. What I found so grotesque about that statement apart from the mutilation of my mother tongue, was the fact that if PGD had been available one generation earlier, she would not have been here to offer up her opinion. She might indeed have the right, after extensive counselling, to decide for herself to go through the rigours and expense of IVF and PGD, but to suggest that the rightness of that decision was self- evident, trivialises the issue.

Now let us try and get to grips with slippery slopes and eugenics. The term "eugenics" was coined by Francis Galton (1822-1911). He was an English scientist who studied heredity and intelligence and happened to be a cousin of Charles Darwin. Erasmus Darwin was Francis Galton's maternal grandfather and also Charles Darwin's paternal grandfather, so Galton was indeed fortunate to have been born into a family whose genetic pool included members of the Wedgwood and Keynes families. Galton defined his new word this way: "Eugenics is the study of agencies under social control that may improve or impair the racial qualities of future generations, whether physically or mentally." In 1905, he wrote about the three stages of eugenics, first an academic matter, then a practical policy, and finally that "it must be introduced into the national consciousness as a new religion." He described his ideas in an article entitled "Hereditary Character and Talent" (published in two parts in *MacMillan's Magazine,* vol. 11, November 1864 and April 1865, pp. 157-166, 318-327), expressing his frustration that no one was breeding a better human race:

> "If a twentieth part of the cost and pains were spent in measures for the improvement of the human race that is spent on the improvement of the breed of horses and cattle, what a galaxy of genius might we not create! We might introduce prophets and high priests of civilization into the world, as surely as we can propagate idiots by mating cretins. Men and women of the present day are, to those we might hope to bring into existence, what the pariah dogs of the streets of an Eastern town are to our own highly-bred varieties."

What is so chilling about reading these ramblings of an old Victorian bigot one hundred years later, is the fact that Adolf Hitler and the third Reich attempted to apply these principles in practice with mass sterilisation of inmates of mental asylums and undesirable non Aryans as a prelude to mass murder.

I'm pretty sure that the HFEA does not have in mind that we should start building a master race of blond, blue eyed, athletic geniuses but is their endorsement of PGD to select out embryos predetermined to develop cancer in young adulthood the first step down a slippery slope towards a Galtonian

Utopia. I think not. For a start I don't subscribe to the "slippery slope" principle in ethics debates. This presupposes that there is a line of ethical principle that must never be crossed that is viewed from a point on the moral high ground. One step down, one concession, one turning of a blind eye and society loses its footing sliding downwards into the ethical abyss. This as you see is argument by analogy. We have already made concessions in selecting babies. For example amniocentesis is commonly used before aborting foetuses with X linked hemophilia or Downs' syndrome. This technique can be abused for sex selection but that abuse, is covered by law. A recent high-profile case in India ended when a gynaecologist who profited by aborting female foetuses was given a stiff jail sentence. No doubt the problem is rife in China where there is a one- child policy but in this example, sex selection is the consequence of social engineering not the reverse.

Furthermore PGD is already available for families bearing the gene for cystic fibrosis, Tay Sachs disease, Huntingdon's chorea and thalasaemia; all dreadful diseases with early age onset. This as far as I know has never been associated with a slide down the slope of ethical compromise. So what makes the new ruling so controversial? In screening embryos for the BRCA mutations that predispose to breast cancer and hereditary polyposis coli (HPC) the word is predispose. In other words not inevitable. For example BRCA2 has about a 50% penetrance for breast cancer and breast cancer can be prevented by prophylactic mastectomy for all cases with BRCA mutations. In the same way colo-rectal cancer can be prevented in HPC by prophylactic colectomy. These are not trivial interventions but have to be weighed up against the very nature of personhood. I can see how PGD could breed out the faulty gene in the fullness of time and spare mothers from the guilt and anxiety of passing it on but I can also understand the argument that you might be destroying an embryo, albeit only eight cells in total, that might lead to an adult of unknown potential who might lead a full and productive life. At the same time I know that left to nature about half such embryos at this stage of gestation would spontaneously abort or as Gillian Lockwood, chairman of the British Fertility Society's ethical committee so eloquently put it; "half the eggs fertilized naturally don't become babies and we are not in a perpetual state of mourning". So can I take a position on this? Well like all of us it's only when it's up front and personal that the hypothetical debate becomes a matter of serious decision- making.

As chance would have it at the very time I was pondering these issues a front -page article appeared in the Daily Telegraph of May 15th entitled "We had to go abroad to get our baby screened". Below that was a lovely family photograph of Dr. Mandy Baum (my niece!), her husband, her oldest son affected with tuberous sclerosis (TS), her second son without the inherited gene and her baby son selected successfully to be free of TS by IVF and PGD at a clinic in Brussels. Of course I knew this was in the offing but the timing was remarkable and when I think back about all the suffering and anguish Mandy and her husband Phillip went through to reach this happy outcome I had no doubt it was the right choice for them.

Last year our family went through another period of crisis when my sister agreed to be tested for a BRCA mutation because of the familial predisposition to breast cancer, for the sake of her four daughters, another clutch of nieces, fortunately she tested negative. Had she had tested positive I don't think I would have wanted the gene bred out of the family because I'm confident that in such cases breast cancer will one day be preventable and in due course curable. Furthermore for all we know breeding out one undesirable gene might be associated with the inadvertent loss of a desirable gene from the same pool. Those are my opinions but in the end the technology is here to stay, it cannot be un-invented and like all technology can be used for good or for evil. What is needed is control and mature debate. It's neither eugenics nor a no brainer.

Chapter 43

The Archaeology of Race

Debbie Challis

Bloomsbury publishers 2013

(Book Review for Palestine Exploration Fund as yet unpublished)

This is a remarkable and captivating book but before I begin my review I thought it might be amusing if I started by explaining how I came to be the reviewer. I'm not an archaeologist but by chance I found myself well qualified for the task as professor emeritus of surgery at University College London (UCL). Having retired from my chair I thought I'd try my hand at writing fiction amongst other things. My first novel, "The Third Tablet of the Holy Covenant" was published on November the first 2013. The central core of the story related to events proximal to the fall of the second Temple in Jerusalem in 70CE. This had been festering away in my head for 50 years ever since I was a freshly minted surgeon volunteering to work for professor Yigal Yadin at the Masada dig. I was bereft on completing that task so I decided to write a sequel linked to events at the time of the fall of King Solomon's Temple in 587 BCE. Whereas I knew quite a bit about the events in 70-73CE from reading Josephus and getting my hands dirty at Masada, I was starting from scratch for my second work of fiction so after a life time researching into cancer I embarked on a new career as an armchair archaeologist. I started with the "Lachish letters" at the British Museum and that lead me to the man JL Starkey. Reading about Starkey's untimely death I learnt that he had been mentored by that great Egyptologist and professor at my own University,

William Flinders Petrie. That then lead to the mystery of his headless body being buried in Jerusalem whilst for reasons beyond my ken, his head was stored somewhere in my very own Royal College of Surgeons (RCS). The archivist at the RCS very kindly searched out the files linked to this bizarre gift and I spent a very instructive hour or two wading through the material. I deduced from the other contents of the file that the recipient of the first letter was Sir Arthur Keith, Hunterian Professor and conservator of the Hunterian Museum of the Royal College of Surgeons in London and I copy an extract below:

Government Hospital, Department of Health
Government of Palestine, Jerusalem
9/10/44

Dear Sir Arthur,

When Sir Flinders Petrie was admitted to the British section of this hospital on 27/10/40 with B.T. malaria at the age of 87, one of the very earliest requests he made in case he should not survive the attack, was that his skull should be sent to the museum of the Royal College of Surgeons under your care as a specimen of a typical British skull

As you know he died on the 28/7/42 and he had more than once reiterated his wish to preserve his skull for you. The night he died, Dr. Krikorian and I removed the head after injecting Muller's solution and to be sure that the solution had been effective in the brain tissue the vault was taken off. It was found that to be well infiltrated and the brain is now preserved in formalin and is available for transfer to you when the occasion is possible to be sent at some future date along with archaeological material when the war is over. The willing and even anxious cooperation of Lady Petrie in this matter forestalled any feelings of desecration.

Yours Faithfully
Dr. W .E. Thompson (specialist)

The next letter, although innocent in content, shocked me by its provenance:

Department of Applied Statistics
University of London, University College
The Francis Galton Eugenics Laboratory The Biometric Laboratory

To Sir Arthur Keith Royal College of Surgeons 19/11/32

Dear Sir Arthur,

Many thanks for your kind letter of congratulations. I admire the generosity of the Germans to an alien enemy more than their wisdom in selecting myself.

Karl Pearson

An academic department of Eugenics at my University!? This must be a shameful and closely guarded secret of the past. The rest of the file contained a three-way exchange of correspondence between Flinders Petrie, Karl Pearson and Sir Arthur Keith discussing "Biometrics" and the statistical proof behind the racist theory of Eugenics. Much of the material from Petrie was written by hand and difficult to read but there was no denying from this evidence that institutionalised racism nested in the very heart of the academic aristocracy in London, infesting my University and my College.

I then embarked on a journey of discovery from the department of Archaeology at UCL where Rachel Sparks proved very helpful, from there to the Petrie Museum and finally to the library and archives of the Palestine Exploration Fund (PEF). At the PEF I was warmly welcomed by Felicity Cobbing, paid my dues and started to work my way through their archive linked to the excavations at Lachish. On my third visit Felicity was holding this book in her hand and rightly guessed that I might be the man to review it. So that in part is my agenda in carrying out this pleasurable duty but a darker agendum became clear as I got deeper into the book.

In the opening chapter, Debbie Challis (Audience development officer at the Petrie museum of Egyptology UCL) makes clear what her agenda was for writing the book and I felt a little foolish in thinking that I had made some kind of original discovery when so much scholarship on the subject was laid out before me.

The author writes as the curator of the exhibition at UCL "Typecast", to mark the centenary of Francis Galton. The opening chapter describes Debbie Challis' struggle to come to terms with the Eugenic theories of Galton and how they were exploited to justify imperialism as the “White man’s burden”. Although not the main thrust of the book she starts off by describing a ghoulish device, *haarfarbentafel,* a gauge for measuring hair colour and texture in the possession of the Petrie museum, that was bought by Karl Pearson from Eugen Fischer, the Director of the Institute of Racial Hygiene in Berlin later appointed by Adolf Hitler as rector of the Frederik Wilhem University in 1933. So at once the circle, that I naively thought I had discovered, was complete, Galton, Pearson, Petrie and some unspeakable villains in Hitler’s inner circle. But that is not the real theme of the book, which is to illustrate how Petrie’s genius as a pioneer in Egyptology was subverted to justify a belief in eugenics, racism and colonialism.

The history of racism starts with Robert Knox, a mid 19th C surgeon in Edinburgh, notorious because of his association with Burke and Hare. His book, "Races of men", expressed negative opinions about Jews and Celts. Challis was disturbed by "objectification" of human remains in the Knox museum at Surgeons Hall in Edinburgh, from person to thing.

Such concerns reappear later in the first chapter when she describes how Knox used human props to illustrate the morphology of “inferior” races in his lectures. At the same time, Morton in the USA published “*Crania Americana*” where he built a racial hierarchy based on phrenology with white Europeans on top and black Africans near bottom.

Such ideas of course were used to support slavery.

Knox looked upon race as species with the *ancient* Greeks being the epitome of species who were replaced in league table by latter day Anglo Saxons. He also considered Jews as a species that were parasitic on other cultures. This dehumanization of Jews as a sub-human species was an adumbration of the first step towards the *holocaust* 100 years later. Not all popular opinion supported these ideas as judged by the correspondence columns in the Manchester Times and Gazette.

The anthropological institute of Great Britain & Ireland was established in the 1870s and was led by Darwinian proponents that included Thomas Huxley and Francis Galton. This gave credence to social Darwinism and the "social surgeons" of the eugenic movement. They supported their beliefs on “race and face” by studying the monuments of Ancient Egypt and Ancient Greece. Thus archaeology and anthropology were united at birth of the two disciplines. The Indian uprising (1856-1857) and the American civil war (1861-65) were both fought over issues of race. In the same period, white settlers wiped out the Tasmanian aborigines as if corroborating the prophecies of the eugenicists. Galton's original ideas of inherited intelligence or genius were not considered outrageous in his days, and are often resurrected in contemporary discourse on nature v nurture. However, taken further to suggest improving the human race by breeding was highly controversial at the time. In a chapter in his book "hereditary genius" (the comparative worth of different races), he concluded that the ancient Athenian race ranked two "grades" higher than his own..."That is as much as our race is above the African Negro". These so called "grades" gave his statistics an illusion of objectivity. Most newspaper reviews were hostile. However, *Nature's review* by Alfred Wallace was favourable and Darwin (sadly) was converted. These three Galton, Wallace and Darwin, expressed concern of the dangers of miscegenation and the purity (supremacy) of British stock. The London Olympic festival of 1866 anticipated the Olympic ideal and the new culture of "muscular Christianity" fed on these ideas. This late 19thC adulation of Hellenism was a forerunner of the Fascist ideals. With this cultural *zeitgeist* established, Flinders Petrie enters the fray. He invented a portable anthropometric kit including a "craniometer" in 1885, assuming that craniometry reflected brain mass and intelligence. Petrie prided himself on his own inheritance of skills, virtues and intelligence and therefore placed himself amongst the chosen ones at the pinnacle of the human race. (At this point I began to understand why he gifted his head as a prime specimen of *homo sapiens* to the RCS.) Petrie Idealised the beauty of female face based on archaeological findings of Greek statuettes, as an expression of the epitome of racial evolution. At this point I parted company from Challis in her commentary. Fashion may change but the symmetry of a beautiful face in every continent of the modern world has been a constant over time and may have an evolutionary advantage. What's really at issue is to suggest physiognomy reflects moral and intellectual status. For example Petrie prided himself in his skill at reading faces and would judge and condemn a man as a criminal type on first impressions. He then made use of these "prodigious skills" after collecting photographs or plaster casts of heads from ancient Egyptian bas-relief frescos and statues to define "ancient races of man". Petrie also gifted 40 skulls to Virchow the most renowned medical scientist of those days and must have been a little put out when Virchow then set about denouncing Nordic mysticism and German ideology of purity and hierarchy of race.

In chapter 5 Challis makes a slight deviation from the main subject to discuss the Greco-Roman portraits on mummies from this period. My personal prejudice as someone who teaches the history of art is that the topic is more of relevance to art history than the history of race theory. I believe that the haunting naturalism of these portraits act as link to bridge the gap between the art of the Classic period and the Renaissance and I was glad to note that Brian Sewell agrees with me after an exhibition of the faces in 1997. However I was amused to learn that Petrie and his followers who plundered these graves, assumed that some of these portraits to be Hellenic Greeks, attractively tanned by the sun rather than "Semitic" types, in order to reinforce their prejudices. “The real pluri-potential of these mummy faces transcends the feeble false science of physiognomy in reading the face”, concludes Challis with her wonderful prose and startlingly original philosophical insights.

The mood then turns darker in a later chapter, “Peopling the Old Testament” where she describes how the advocates of morphometrics accounted for the degeneration of the Jewish race *(sic)* as demonstrated by the "ghetto expression" of the Semitic features described in Galton's composite photos. All this has been objectively refuted by recent discoveries concerning the molecular genealogy of the Jewish people, an example of which is the discovery of the Cohen model haplotype on the Y chromosome as described by Neil Bradman at University College London.

In a masterful act of convoluted thinking Petrie and his fellow travellers eventually arrived at the belief that the Virgin Mary was of European stock and that Joseph the Jew was not really the father of Jesus and that somehow or other justified the British mandate in Palestine!

Galton et al could have never guessed the long-term terrible unintended consequences of their work at the time of the Nazis, yet Cultural racism as a justification for colonial appropriation has left scars to this day in post-colonial Africa and Middle East. Such prejudices even led to claims that the Great Zimbabwe was beyond the skills of Negroid Africans but had been built by a superior race in the distant past. As a *reductio ad absurdum* Petrie then went on to postulate a migrant race in pre-dynastic times to account for the achievements of the greatest civilization of the Iron Age. This preposterous concept was fuelled by morphometric analysis of skulls from Naqada and statistical advice from Pearson sitting in comfort at the Galton laboratory of Eugenics at UCL. Petrie even used this belief to support the colonialist ideology of not offering the natives an education beyond their racial capacity. Petrie politics were fully developed in his book *Janus in modern life* 1907, a eugenics manifesto. He objected to reforms on child welfare that favoured nurture over nature as a way of overcoming poverty and low expectations of life.

His most repugnant view was to dismiss the poor as being the "worst stock" and the urban poor almost looked upon as a separate race, using the expression "weeding out inferior stock”.

Overall I find Petrie a repulsive man even if judged by the standards of the time. My grandparents would have been weeded out for sure as the "lowest types of immigrants from Poland" (Petrie's own words). My late brother David died in office as President of the Royal College of Paediatrics, my older brother Harold completed his career as Dean of life Science at Kings College London and the next generation of my family can already boast four professors in the life sciences. This is the living proof that social justice in a liberal democracy has more to offer than the pseudoscientific claptrap of eugenics. There-I've gone and said it. That was the other darker agenda I hinted at earlier, with which I approached this magisterial book.

Chapter 44

Back to the Future

(Editorial, International J Surgery, 2012;10, 3 - 4.)

I recently saw the film, “Midnight in Paris”, a work of genius by Woody Allan. In this story a young American writer visiting Paris shortly before his wedding, becomes besotted by the beauty and history of the city. He then imagines what it must have been like in the heady days of the 1920s. To him this was the “golden era” of literary and artistic endeavor. The twist in the tale is when our hero experiences time travel at the stroke of midnight when he is picked up from the steps of a bridge over the Seine by a limousine dating from the 1920s.

To his amazement the plush interior is peopled by some of his heroes of the Jazz age. Immediately he is plunged into the golden era of his dreams, where he meets luminaries such as Scott Fitzgerald, Gertrude Stein, Cole Porter, Picasso, Salvador Dali, and best of all Ernest Hemingway. He finds himself competing for the affections of the beautiful young ingénue who is both the mistress of the Picasso and Hemingway. When he returns to the present day of course no one believes his story and a pedantic and scholarly acquaintance of his fiancé points out there that there never was a “golden era” and that he mustn't forget about how many of these beautiful young things were struck down by tuberculosis before their time.

The Past

I was thinking of this film when I sat down to write this little piece about the past, present and the future of information technology (IT) and scholarly publication. The first thing I was reminded of was the cautionary note that there never was a golden age. I qualified in 1960 and, shortly after gaining my FRCS, embarked on a career in cancer research. My FRCS certificate hanging by my desk carries the names of the surgical luminaries of that era that include, Lord Brock, Sir Hedley Atkins, Eastcote and Naughton Morgan. There was no IT in those days. Furthermore I had to do mathematical calculations for statistical analysis on a slide rule rather than a computer. I remember hours and hours spent in dusty libraries searching back volumes with the help of Index Medicus, each volume of which weighed about 7 kg. What little aid the librarians could provide for me consisted of long drawers in huge mahogany chests that contained thousands of index cards cross-referenced by author and topic. My interest at the time was related to the immune response to cancer and its potential for the development of immunotherapy. For that reason I had to closely monitor a host of journals that included the New England Journal of Medicine, the Lancet, BMJ, Cancer, Cancer Research, Science, Nature, and any other journal that contained cancer or immunology in its title. As I followed these journals I would take notes of the important papers and transcribe them onto index cards. For those journals that I received by my subscriptions, I would tear out the pages to keep in box files in addition to adding my notes to the growing pile of index cards. These index cards then had to be cross referenced in the same way as the library into miniature versions of the mahogany chest of drawers in the dusty libraries which turned out to be cardboard boxes in my dusty study at home. When I say, “study”, I'm really joking at my own expense, at the very best it was a corner of the kitchen table or a corner of my wife’s vanity table in the bedroom.

Far worse than data gathering was the data retrieval when I started to write up research papers and subsequently write up my thesis, trying to retrieve key references from my boxes of cards or my files of the original papers. By the time I became professor of surgery at Kings in 1980, I had built up a library of references that filled up 60 or 70 box files. These box files then filled up most of the available bookcase shelving in my office in the Department of surgery. Fortunately I was able to dispose of all my files a year ago when out of the blue, the University of Wales Cardiff, requested my archive for the historical section of their library. I was deeply flattered that at least one university thought that some Ph.D. student in the distant future, using the latest IT technology, would be able to discover all the mistakes I have made in the past, directing research in the wrong direction. Of course I secretly hope that this hypothetical Ph.D. student in the future might encounter the rare occasions where I had set a fertile agenda for the next generation.

The Present

Now in my latest incarnation as professor emeritus of surgery at University College London, I have a lovely study in my house as well as an office in my department, where I'm still actively involved in directing large-scale multi centre clinical trials. Both my offices are virtually paperless and to my own amazement I'm dictating this article to my Apple Mac computer entirely by voice recognition. As well as saving me time in typing with one finger, the voice recognition system has more skill in spelling than I have. Even when I'm typing with Microsoft "Word", the software cannot begin to guess the word I have misspelled; I think to some extent I'm mildly dyslexic.

Using the latest IT techniques, all the papers I've read are saved as PDF files and these files organized into folders on my desktop window or saved in a very easily traceable way on my hard drive. Even if I forget the title of the file I'm looking for, all I need to do is type a few search words into the "spotlight" panel at the top right hand corner of my screen and a drop-down menu will find the paper or the reference, in seconds. I do still like to be surrounded by books in spite of having a paperless office. But now that I have iPad 2 I'm at a point of equipoise regarding whether I prefer hard copy in a beautifully bound volume or softcopy downloaded in a matter of minutes to my tablet.

However, speaking as a clinical scientist, the biggest advantage I enjoy from exploiting the latest in IT, is the ease of access to the totality of the medical literature in all languages in all countries of the world. I have a number of search engines that I subscribe to, where in a matter of minutes I can trace any article by any author on any topic published anywhere in the world. Furthermore I no longer need to monitor the content pages of these leading journals covering my field. Others do this for me. They may be real people who are aware of my interest or belong to the same Google group with common interests, who keep me up to date by e-mail. They may also be angels floating out there in cyberspace, dredging the cloud of digital data to identify topics of great interest to the humanoid, Prof M Baum, and then distilling the information and zoning it directly to my desktop computer. Sadly, a consequence of all this is that I rarely visit an actual rather than virtual library. I still love the atmosphere of scholarship when I enter an old dusty mahogany walled library, with intense young students beavering away at their desks. Even that image is fading fast as the desks in the libraries that I visit nowadays at University College or the Royal Free, not to mention my favorite library at the Royal Society of Medicine, are mahogany free and mostly taken up by computers like my own, rather than by pyramids of books. Probably the one thing I miss most of all is the "library gremlin". Very few of you reading this article would understand what this means; it's a generational thing. The "library gremlin" describes the chance event when you were searching the stacks for one volume of one journal and accidentally knock down a volume from another shelf that randomly opens at page where, to your amazement something central to your line of investigation is found entirely by chance. This is the work of a gremlin that is never seen but that we can imagine to be giggling quietly to itself, in some dusty corner of the bookshelf.

The Future

Coming back now to the hypothetical Ph.D. student 20 years from now who decides to search the archive of the University of Wales to try and find out something about the history of breast cancer research and has happened upon my name, I actually have difficulty in projecting my thoughts into this distant future because, as far as I'm concerned I'm really living in the "golden age" of IT. Of course it's not tuberculosis that I'm worried about but rather the computer virus that might creep up on me and wipe out my hard drive. In the short time I've been involved with the International Journal of Surgery it's already become paperless and "Wikkified". How much better can it get? Well I suppose one step forward relates to the fact that that I'm talking to my computer without men in white coats coming to carry me back to the asylum. Recently my daughter-in-law demonstrated a new iPhone 4, which responds to voice commands. It is easy to predict therefore, that a Ph.D. student in the future will simply sit down at his or her desk and say to the iPhone 7* "fetch me all the records related to endocrine therapy of breast cancer with Baum as one of the authors in the period 1980 to 1990. Please sort out the wheat from chaff": and suddenly it would all appear on the screen that is embedded in their wristwatch and from there projected onto any convenient whitewall. I'm not serious about that last stuff, I can't think of anything worse. We mustn't forget that part of scholarship and reflective thinking involves sitting in a comfortable space of your own, free from noise and distraction. I cannot imagine a time in the future where this will cease to be important.

In fact, in projecting the future, I think I've made a fundamental mistake in assuming that knowledge will continue to grow exponentially and that all this knowledge will be of equal value. I fondly predict that the speed at which new data is collected and disseminated will slow down as a consequence of checks on the quality of information that is being delivered to the learned journals. Already we are seeing checks and balances in the method of peer review and that's something else I acknowledge as part of the progress in IT.

Please slow the pace of innovation; I'm comfortable in this anchorage for a while.

Chapter 45

Valedictory Editorial for the International Journal of Surgery

International Journal of Surgery
Volume 4, Issue 4, Pages 197–198, 2006

As I find myself half way through my 70th year on this planet and as I will be shortly celebrating the 45th year as a registered doctor with my surviving classmates from Birmingham University School of Medicine, I thought it time to hang up my editorial hat and pass it on to someone younger and better in touch with our global surgical brotherhood/sisterhood. That last minute addition of sisterhood must tell you something. When I gained my Fellowship of the Royal College of Surgeons of England (FRCS) in 1965 there were no female fellows in my group whereas today I'm delighted to note that about half of our new FRCSs carry two X chromosomes. It is therefore appropriate for me to reflect on the changes I've witnessed in the practice of surgery in the last 40 years before I enter my "anecdotage".

Apart from all these bright young women bustling about the place there have been many obvious and equally glamorous developments in surgical techniques. Transplantation, minimally invasive surgery and interventional radiology immediately come to mind. In parallel with that have been the breathtaking breakthroughs in diagnostic imaging such as fibre-optic flexible endoscopy, CT and MRI scans. Of course along the way the invention of drugs such as the H2 receptor antagonists and antimicrobial therapy for peptic ulcers (two Nobel prizes here) has led to the loss of much of the upper GI surgery that occupied nearly half of my general surgical lists in the late 1960s and early 1970s. Advances in trauma surgery, led by the doctors in the front line of civil unrest or outright war, have changed the face of the A&E departments and intensive care lead by our colleagues in the anaesthetic departments, continues to salvage victims of major injury or burns, who most certainly would have died in the first decade after I qualified.

Surgical research has flourished and academic departments of surgery burgeoned in number, reaching a peak in the 1990s, but are now facing what looks like a terminal decline *(vide infra).* By surgical research I don't just mean research into surgical technique, but a much broader definition, as research into disease that is commonly referred to surgeons. Surgeons have lead the way in randomised controlled trials even though the outcome of these trials has led to a reduction in the number of surgical interventions in use, as exemplified above. Audit has emerged as an essential component of our everyday life and the ethics of our interactions with our patients has been researched and codified in a number of surgical textbooks.

But...something of immense value has been lost along the way. "Oh dear", I can hear you murmur behind your hands, "Baum's going to talk about the Good Old Days!". Well to an extent that's true. I think the trajectory of my experience as a surgeon has described a parabola with something like a golden age in the late 1970s until the early 1990s that applies not to only the research ethos but also to professionalism as a whole. I don't completely blame the constant re-disorganization of the National Health Service (NHS) or the European Union (EU) attempts at harmonization; I also blame some of our younger colleagues for allowing it to happen. Sure, when I qualified, any time off was considered a rare privilege, not a right, and a lot of the time we were wickedly exploited propping up the NHS whilst our chiefs got on with the serious business of making money in the private sector. However, one thing of lasting value we learnt was the sense of total open-ended responsibility and continuity of care for the sick and the lame assigned to our watch. I will never forget the sense of guilt I felt when I was off duty and one of my charges developed complications or, God forbid, had to be re-operated on by another surgeon. This is what I mean by professionalism; an open ended contract.

Thanks to cost cutting in the NHS and the malign interventions of the EU we have gone to another extreme. Hours are so tightly controlled that many junior doctors are not indemnified to even being on the premises of their hospital once they've completed their set time on duty. Furthermore, audit and clinical governance activities count towards their hours of duty, leaving less time for work and experience on the front line. Add to that shift work, annual leave, paternity/maternity leave, compassionate leave and study leave, no one seems to be left in charge, all that at a time when I enter the age bracket that may well need the skills and attention of a youthful surgeon.

You may think that these ideas are old fashioned and reactionary and that a proper work life balance is equally as important as professional responsibility. Well I confess I do subscribe to some pretty old-fashioned ideas that include politeness, chivalry, a work ethic and the constant need for reflection and research that goes on out of hours.

Well, the chickens have come home to roost. It is increasingly difficult to recruit academic surgeons, as time out for research interferes with the mechanics of the sausage machine that turns out surgical functionaries that will fulfil the EU requirements for specialist status. In addition, academic departments of surgery are closing down or being subsumed into larger amorphous entities of life science research. One of the most bittersweet moments of this year was when I was asked to speak at the *Festschrift* for one of my academic colleagues left over from my days as Professor of Surgery at Kings College School of Medicine and Dentistry. In those days we had three professors, three senior lecturers, umpteen lecturers and clinical research fellows but he was the last. His retirement ended the line of a distinguished academic unit that started with Lord Lister in 1908 and ended with a whimper as the last one to leave turned off the lights.

Ahh! I feel better for that rant which I found quite cathartic. I wish the journal a great future under new leadership but I will still keep a close eye on things in my role as Emeritus Editor in Chief.

Chapter 46

The Meaning of Life and Other Easy Questions

(First written for a book celebrating the 150th anniversary of the Red Cross but greatly expanded and published in my memoires "Breast Beating: A personal Odyssey in the quest for an understanding of breast cancer, the meaning of life and other easy questions" Publishers Anshan Ltd, Tunbridge Wells, 2010, reprinted by kind permission of the publishers)

> "Tomorrow and tomorrow and tomorrow creeps in this petty pace from day to day to the last syllable of recorded time and all our yesterdays have lighted fools the way to dusty death. Out, out brief candle! Life's but a walking shadow. A poor player that struts and frets his hour upon the stage until he is heard no more. It is a tale told by an idiot full of sound and fury signifying nothing."
>
> Macbeth, Act V, Scene V.

I learnt this soliloquy from Macbeth by heart, at about the age of seven and used it as my "party piece" whenever my parents had the opportunity to show off their gifted children in front of an appreciative audience of family and friends. What my parents could never have predicted was the consequence of my sudden understanding of this bleak passage, when at about the age of eleven, I embarked on my lifelong career as a professional insomniac. I remember clearly as a precocious young boy, lying awake all night trying to determine which was worse, to live forever, or to die at some uncertain point in the future and what was life all about anyway? Shakespeare's suggestion that it signified nothing added a new layer or terror to my troubled nights. However, with the passage of time my experience of life (and for that matter my experience of death), I think I've been able to define the questions with considerably more maturity than that of the pre-pubescent lad. I therefore welcome the opportunity this publication provides me with, to try to synthesize fifty years of self-questioning as to the meaning of life and the relevance of this to my clinical practice.

My attitude to the big question has been shaped by three major influences. These influences have been, my upbringing as a Jew, my scientific curiosity as a practicing clinical scientist and my lifelong passionate affair with the visual arts. I don't think it's any exaggeration or particular conceit to say that sometimes I have to draw on all these inner resources in counseling my patients to help them make difficult decisions that might influence both the length and quality of their lives.

In the quiet doldrums between Christmas and the end of the New Year holiday break in 1995, I was called in to help a young woman make one of the toughest choices that anyone can ever be called upon to decide.

In fact the decision reminded me of “Sophie’s choice” in William Styron’s tragic novel of the same name.

A Case History

The young woman in question was a pretty Greek Orthodox girl aged thirty-one. Four years earlier she had been diagnosed with breast cancer at a time when she was twelve weeks pregnant. The pregnancy was terminated and she underwent a conventional course of treatment that involved surgery, radiotherapy and chemotherapy. She was very keen to start a family and I advised her to wait a year or two. It should be noted in passing that a pregnancy after breast cancer has been treated does not influence the prognosis, contrary to popular myth. At the time I was called in to advise, she was twenty -one weeks pregnant and had already felt the quickening of the baby in her womb. Tragically, she had also felt the symptoms of the secondary cancer in her spine. In addition to the severe pain that she experienced, she also described numbness and paresis affecting her left arm. Investigations demonstrated that there were secondaries in the spine, compressing the spinal cord and the nerve roots to her left arm. The various therapeutic options we had to consider included surgery for immediate decompression of the spinal cord, radiotherapy to the vertebra and cytotoxic chemotherapy. To do nothing at that stage would have been unthinkable as without treatment she would have become paraplegic in about 48 hours. Yet, the most effective treatments to prevent this dreaded complication and to add to the length and quality to her remaining life, would compromise the health or viability of the baby in the womb. Whose life was of greater value and whose decision was it anyway? Was the potential life of the unborn more meaningful than prolonging the life of a young adult? I was hoping that her own religious beliefs would guide me in this tough decision, but when asked directly she confessed to being a lapsed Christian and asked me for all the facts so that she could make an informed choice. Amongst the difficult truths that I had to convey was the fact that with even the best of all treatments her expectation of life would be unlikely to exceed two years and therefore should she allow a new life into the world the baby would grow up motherless. There was clearly no correct answer to this dilemma and I will return to the conclusion of this sad story at the end of the chapter.

Judaic Influences

All we know for sure is this life and the history of other lives. Life after death is purely speculative and Jews do not believe that this life is a preparation for the afterlife. Yet in spite of that, there is an almost unspoken assumption amongst Jews that they will be rewarded for a virtuous life, after death. For example, the prayer in the house of mourning: *"Have mercy upon her. Pardon all her transgressions for there is none righteous upon the earth who doeth only good and sinneth not. Remember unto her the righteousness that she wrought and let her reward be with her and her recompense before him - bestow upon her the abounding happiness that is treasured up for the righteous".* And yet paradoxically, on leaving the house of mourning our greeting to the principle mourners is to wish them a long life. We believe that life is of infinite worth and as infinity cannot be split then every moment of a life is of infinite value. We are therefore commanded to strive to preserve and prolong life and to avoid hazardous activities that risk our lives (and that should include smoking). This also explains our contempt for the suicide bombers, those who send them on their way and those who worship them as martyrs.

There are of course, some mystical Chasidic sects who wish to explore the meaning of life and speculate on the afterlife, but mainstream Judaism accepts life as an end in itself and our religious teachings are primarily aimed at providing a code of conduct with more attention being paid to the relationships between man and man than between man and his God. Even to question whether life has a meaning may be a meaningless question to a Jew. If life is an end in itself then to question its meaning is as empty an exercise as to question the meaning of virtue, truth and beauty. With our essential belief in an omnipotent and omniscient God all else follows. If there is a meaning to life then it has to be beyond our comprehension however many subtle clues may pass across our consciousness. We are analogous to the fish trying to comprehend life on earth when all its fish-like brain can perceive are distorted two-dimensional images that appear in its firmament. I would even go further and suggest it is the ultimate in intellectual arrogance to "know" the answer to this question. I happen to note that there is a tendency amongst those who "know" with certainty, to impose their beliefs on others and this in my opinion is the source of most of the world's problems. This confident knowledge of the unknowable leads to religious fundamentalism, forced conversion, terrorism and the three horsemen of the apocalypse.

The Teachings of Biological Science

It is natural for human beings to see patterns in their life. For every effect they like to know the cause. For example, is cancer a punishment? Is it a fault of lifestyle? Is it in the family? Why me? For every patient therefore, there is an emotional need to understand a little about the nature of cancer if only to remove the guilt and the stigma, which has been associated with it in the past. The aetiology of cancer probably involves two basic steps: *initiation,* which may be a necessary but not sufficient cause, and a second set of events, which are described as *promotional.* Apart from the rare cases of genetic predisposition to cancer, initiating factors are exogenous (from without) whereas promotional factors are largely constitutional (from within). There are some obvious examples where clearly defined exogenous factors initiate the disease and where in theory prevention is possible. The best example of course is smoking and its impact on the incidence of lung cancer, bladder cancer and head and neck cancer. Another well established example of this kind is the association between malignant melanoma of the skin and the exposure of white races to excessive sunlight. It is likely that the initiation of the majority of common and for that matter, uncommon cancers are random events resulting from exogenous factors beyond our control leading to somatic mutations in the human genome. These may result from cosmic rays, radon from the granite of the earth or the low, persistent background of x-radiation. We assume that there are constant random mutations occurring within our genome, but we have exquisite repair mechanisms and to an extent our vulnerability to cancer may not be so much due to the exogenous factors as to inherent failures of our natural repair mechanisms. Our new understanding of molecular biology describes what are known as proto-oncogenes, anti-oncogenes and their mechanism of action. We can now begin to understand how random mutations can activate a proto-oncogene into an oncogene, which then instructs the cell in the mechanisms of immortality and metastatic spread.

Alternatively, the genetic damage can knock out an anti-oncogene, which naturally controls these unwelcome properties within an individual cell. We are thus rapidly developing a mechanistic concept of the nature of cancer, which will ultimately lead to rational biological cures. In the meantime, we have to ask whether this increasing knowledge can help us understand cancer from the humanistic point of view. How can a cancer doctor retain any semblance of faith, which is tested each time he witnesses the suffering imposed by this dreadful disease. Paradoxically, each time I contemplate the micro-cosmos of the cancer cell, I find my faith restored. Of course it is commonplace to see God's work in the cosmos as illustrated by the last paragraph of Stephen Hawking's best seller "A Brief History of Time": *"There may be only one complete unified theory that is self-consistent and allow the existence of structures as complicated as human beings who can investigate the laws of the universe and ask about the nature of God. If we find the answer to that, it would be the ultimate triumph of human reason, for then we would know the mind of God*". I enjoy the same sense of awe from the study of inner space rather than outer space. Watson and Crick discovered the structure of DNA in 1953 and subsequent biological scientists have come up with mind-boggling statistics as awe inspiring as those related to cosmology. Richard Dawkins puts it this way. There are 3×10^{12} cells in the body and 46 chromosomes per cell. 2 meters of DNA are packed into the nucleus of each cell tightly wound on these chromosomes. That is 6×10^{12} meters of DNA in each body, which is equivalent to the distance to the moon and back 8000 times! Each time the cell divides there is the hazard of a somatic mutation as a random event. Some cells divide every 48 hours. It is therefore a miracle to me that life can be sustained at all and the question "why me?" whenever someone develops cancer should be turned on its head and every day of everyone's life we should offer up a prayer to thank God that we *didn't* develop cancer in the previous 24 hours. Richard Dawkins in his most readable and mischievous book "The Blind Watchmaker" describes the fidelity of the transcription process beautifully and I wish to quote one of his passages at length: "DNA's performance as an archival medium is spectacular. In its capacity to preserve a message it far outdoes tablets of stone. Letters carved on gravestones become unreadable in mere hundreds of years. The DNA document is even more impressive, because unlike tablets of stone it is not the same physical structure that lasts and preserves the text. It is repeatedly being copied and recopied as the generations go by, like the Hebrew Scriptures, which were ritually copied by scribes every eighty years to forestall their wearing out. It is hard to estimate how many times the DNA document has been recopied in our lineage; probably as many as twenty billion times. It is hard to find a yardstick with which to compare the preservation of more than 99% of the information in twenty billion successive copying."

Such precision is miraculous. Life in the first place is miraculous and preservation of our species is miraculous. Cancer is the inevitable result of any instability within the human genome without which evolution would have been postponed. Cancer therefore is the inevitable result of the gift of life and the evolution of a species to its current state of self-awareness that allows it to ask such questions. We should therefore give thanks for this gift however brief the candle within our grasp. One could therefore say that in asking the question "What is the meaning of life?" we are effectively looking a gift horse in the mouth. It could then be argued why have I been wasting my time as a surgical oncologist?

I have given you the biologist's reason to believe, which includes a belief in reason but I also believe in something transcendental which encourages me to challenge nature.

Lessons from the Study of Fine Art

If life is a miracle, a gift and an end in itself, how do we judge a good life and for how long should we try to extend that life? It is to address these fundamental questions that I have to turn to the arts for guidance. Great works of art, whether they be paintings, music or literature are judged by their capacity to illustrate, interpret and enhance life's experience. I would like to take this definition and use fine art itself as the metaphor to set the parameters for a good and appropriately lengthy life. When judging a great painting I look for harmony of composition, balance of colour and tone and its capacity to evoke emotions of joy or understanding, but even someone unschooled in the appreciation of fine art can recognize an unfinished work when he sees it. For example, Leonardo da Vinci's Adoration of the Kings in the Uffizi Gallery, Florence: this has perfect composition and perspective and certain areas are beautifully sketched in, namely the heads of the Magi and some rearing horses in the distance, yet it is clearly unfinished. Apart from areas of ground color there is little else to give it depth or please the eye with harmony of hue. One despairs of so many of Leonardo's works that remain unfinished as tributes to his flawed genius.

I believe life should be worked upon as with any other expression of the human craving to produce perfection. A good life can be judged at any one time by its horizontal harmonies judged by relationships with family and friends, satisfaction with work or professional advancement and the capacity to enjoy leisure and recreation. Looking at life vertically, a complete and balanced composition would include a time for childhood games, a time for education, a time for marriage and homebuilding, a time for the conception and raising of children, a time to hand over to the next generation, to retire and enjoy the fruits of one's labor and finally a time for a dignified death. Not all of us are capable of creating great works of art, but there is an art in the striving for achievement and even a tragically foreshortened life can leave beauty behind like an unfinished symphony.

My Brother David

Let me tell you about my brother David. He was youngest of the four brothers Baum. He had a lean and hungry look crowned by a huge head of curly hair that made one think of Harpo Marx. He wore exuberant bow ties, did magic and was a deeply religious Jew, indeed a "*Shomer Shabbat*" (Literally guardian of the Sabbath). In contrast I am portly and balding, I wear normal ties and respect those laws of the Sabbath that suit me. We came from the same genetic pool but were of different phenotypes and yet our brains seemed to have been hard- wired in the same way. He was not only a clinical scientist but also a pediatrician. He was a fanatically hard worker and set the pace when we used to study together as undergraduates and registrars in Birmingham.

I couldn't keep up the pace whilst he won all the prizes and the gold medal of his year. He later became professor of Child Heath at the University of Bristol and President of the Royal College of Pediatrics and Child Health. He died whilst leading a charity bike ride to raise money for the children of

Kosovo. He literally and figuratively died in the saddle at the age of 59. He left behind him his wife Angela, an artist and four wonderful boys, Benjamin (Buzz), Joshua, Jacob and Samuel. It was only at his memorial service in Bristol attended by thousands, did I learn of all his achievements in promoting children's health around the globe and the promotion of the hospice movement for children dying from cancer. He combined a zeal for life fueled by his faith and his candle burnt out prematurely flaming at both ends. But what a life, a masterpiece of a life, a life full of color and perfect symmetry yet in many ways an unfinished symphony of a life. He never lived to enjoy that golden retirement he dreamed of, with him studying Talmud in Sefad with Angela painting by his side. The nearest he came to that was his burial plot in Rosh Pinah overlooking his beloved Kineret (The Sea of Galilee). Yet in his for-shortened life he achieved more than most could achieve if they lived to be 120.

The Rajastani Potter

In October 1994, my wife and I visited India to take in the UICC World Cancer Congress in New Delhi. We took advantage of this visit to enjoy a very comfortable and spectacular tour of the Golden Triangle in Rajasthan. On this visit I learnt that of the population of India, which numbers approximately nine hundred million, seven hundred and fifty million live in abject poverty with a life expectancy thirty years less than our own. One cannot possibly begin to imagine the enormity of such numbers and once again it is necessary in order to gain the slightest of insights to focus in on the life of a single individual. We enjoyed three magnificent days staying in the lap of luxury in the Lake Palace Hotel in Udaipur. On one of these days our guide took us through the hills and jungle north of Udaipur to visit the Jain Temples of Ranakpur. Along the way he made a diversion so that we could visit a small rural village where he was well known. Stopping at the side of a rutted and primitive road we continued our journey on foot through all kinds of excreta and rubbish past stagnant pools where the colorful women of Rajasthan were beating their saris clean; through a tumbledown village of mud-bricks and collapsing thatch to a little shed to watch the potter at his work. As always, I enjoyed the creation of an artifact out of formless clay. The potter enjoyed our interest and his wife and countless children were thrilled by the visit of alien creatures from what might have been another planet. Their interest and amusement with us, and the offers of hospitality were disarmingly genuine.

This seemed to be a man, happy with the weft of his life strengthened by his family network and the beauty and utility of the objects he was creating. Also, from what I learned during my visit to India, Hindu festivals and rituals punctuated the warp of his life. Like many of the poor and uneducated in India, he was blissfully unaware of the alternative lifestyle enjoyed by us Westerners and so probably lacked the ambition to "improve himself" and had no desire for consumer durables or skiing holidays. I am well aware that it is easy to romanticize this squalor and look upon this harmless man as a "noble savage", but just as we should try and improve on nature with finding a cure for cancer I believe it should be an expression of our humanity to improve upon nurture so that the health and welfare of this family could be improved. I cannot believe that his life would lose much of value if all his children had a good education and were able to realize their full potential and enjoy the artistic traditions of their own society. I don't believe anything of value would be lost by trying to reduce the appalling infant mortality by the simple expedient of providing fresh, uncontaminated running water and I cannot believe that much of value would be lost if the potter lived long enough to enjoy his grandchildren. This then leaves me with a troubling thought. Would India, or for that matter the rest of the world, be a better place if there were fewer citizens with more complete lives? In other words is birth control and easy access to abortion the only answers to these questions? I certainly don't side with the pro- life fanatics in the United States of America. I can think of no greater obscenity than those who commit murder in the name of the unborn. I tend to side with the sardonic political commentator P J O'Rourke. In his book "All the Worlds Troubles" he points out with devastating logic that population density per se is not the cause of poverty and misery and emphasizes that certain areas of Southern California have a greater population density than the Delta area of Bangladesh. His explanation for the cause of poverty, misery and a high infant mortality is the direct correlation of these world troubles with nations that practice religious intolerance, feudalism and corruption.

Returning now to my metaphor of the weft and warp of life. I recognize that to describe life as a rich tapestry is a rather exhausted cliché, but it will serve my purpose now. A character in Somerset Maugham's lovely fable "A Moon and Sixpence", someone who is clearly a prototype hippy, carries with him at all times a rolled up Persian carpet. He uses this as a "memento vitae". It had always been my ambition to emulate this character and one of the other great successes of our visit to India was to bring back a silken Kashmiri carpet. Due to some brilliant bargaining on behalf of my wife we were able to purchase this exquisite work of art at barely twice that it cost the vendor! Like all true Kashmiri silk carpets it is indeed magic. Viewed from my current position at my writing desk I can enjoy its robust and intricate patterns suggestive of the mathematics of a complex organism. The colors are vivid, rich and dark. Viewed from the other side, it takes on an entirely different character. The shades are pastel, the outlines of the design ephemeral and the carpet appears to float above the ground. Give me my current perspective of this carpet any day and let the metaphysicians enjoy the alternative viewpoint as much as they like, providing they don't impose their view of life on me by forced conversion, torture or decree.

Returning to the Case in Point

Let me now return to the case of the young woman twenty-one weeks' pregnant with impending spinal cord compression from metastatic breast cancer. As an informed and carefully calculated choice she allowed the pregnancy to go to thirty-two weeks before delivery through Caesarean section. This compromise allowed a new life into the world with an almost 100% chance of survival in health to adult life. This child is a reminder to her husband of his late wife. This child will allow a beautiful symmetry in her foreshortened life, denied on the previous occasion at the time of her initial diagnosis. I supported her in this decision from my own ethical standpoint because I was not actively shortening her life for the benefit of the child. This new life started at a disadvantage because of the limited life expectancy of the mother, but the starting point for all works of art are of an infinite variety and what could be a less promising subject than say Van Gough's shoes? Although as a Jew I will always value the life of a mother over the potential life of a foetus, I can recognize the persuasiveness of the argument that a potential life may be valued equally with the fully developed life of the adult.

Envoi

In 1984 I suffered a severe bout of clinical depression. Only fellow sufferers will fully appreciate what this means. It is not simply a sensation of being down in the dumps or thoroughly pissed off with things, but a sense of utter worthlessness and bleak despair. This sensation is certainly illustrated in the passage from Macbeth quoted at the start of this chapter. No amount of reassurance from my family or friends could persuade me that I was of any worth and that my life had any meaning. Towards the end of this illness I experienced an episode that can only be described as a sunburst of happiness and in a crude attempt to emulate Van Gogh I described this feeling with a painting of sunflowers created with a palate knife and thick impasto. Although frightful at that time I think that period of illness was of enormous and lasting value to me. Many people live their life taking it for granted without truly valuing the gift. There is no better way of describing my attitude to life than by using the words of George Bernard Shaw whose feelings are the complete antithesis to those Shakespeare expressed through the mouth of Macbeth:

> "This is the true joy in life, the being used for a purpose recognized by yourself as a mighty one, the being a force of nature instead of a feverish little clod of ailments and grievances complaining that the world will not devote itself to making you happy. I am of the opinion that my life belongs to the whole community, and as long as I live it is my privilege to do for it whatever I can. I want to be thoroughly used up when I die, for the harder I work the more I live. I rejoice in life for its own sake. Life is no brief candle to me. It is a sort of splendid torch which I have got hold of for the moment and I want to make it burn as brightly as possible before handing it on to future generations."

That was how my brother David lived his life and thus was the manner of his parting.

****

Chapter 47

Why me?

(A poem written for a booklet edited by Rabbi Dr. Jeffrey Cohen to provide comfort and amusement for seriously sick patients in hospitals)

Why not me? Let my cells explain,
"Our DNA in double chain,
Replicates a million ways
Each one risks the threads to fray.
Yet God's creative energy
Ensures the gene's heredity."

Why life? The question we should ask.
Yet leave researchers to their task,
Once understood the cancer's claw
Will then explain the natural law,
That all things by our Lord's decree,
Give reason for fidelity.

Acknowledgment

I wish to thank Mrs Hazel Thornton, a doughty patient's advocate, for her loyal support over 20 years of collaboration and for her time and patience in proof reading this work

Author's Contact Information

Dr. Michael Baum
Professor
University College London
Email: Michael@mbaum.freeserve.co.uk
Twitter@MichaelBaum11

Index

#

A

B

D

E

G

H

I

J

K

L

M

Q

R

S

T

U

V

W

X

Y

Z